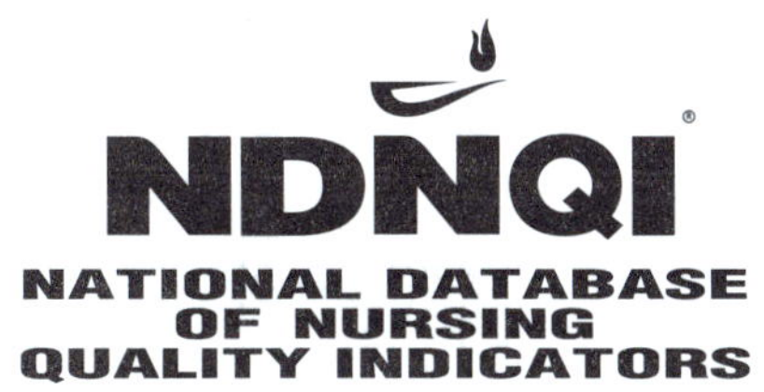

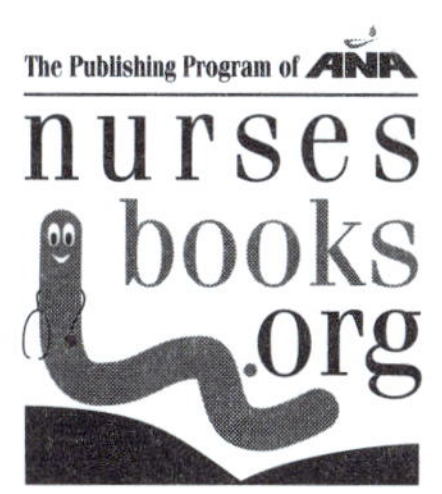

Sustained Improvement in Nursing Quality:

Hospital Performance on NDNQI Indicators, 2007–2008

Nancy Dunton, PhD
Isis Montalvo, RN, MS, MBA
Editors

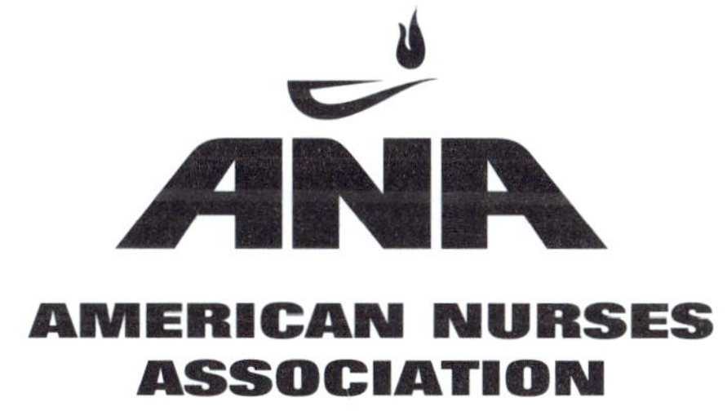

SILVER SPRING, MARYLAND
2009

Library of Congress Cataloging-in-Publication data
Sustained improvement in nursing quality : hospital performance on NDNQI indicators, 2007-2008/ Nancy Dunton and Isis Montalvo, editors.
p. ; cm.
Includes bibliographical references.
ISBN-13: 978-1-55810-264-4 (pbk.)
ISBN-10: 1-55810-264-7 (pbk.)
1. Nursing–United States–Quality control. 2. Hospitals–United States–Quality control.
I. Dunton, Nancy. II. Montalvo, Isis. III. American Nurses Association.
[DNLM: 1. Nursing Process–United States. 2. Quality Indicators, Health Care–United States.
3. Health Facilities–United States. 4. Quality Assurance, Health Care–standards–United States. WY 100 T772 2009]

RT85.5.T73 2009
610.73068–dc24 2009001440

The opinions in this book reflect those of the authors and do not necessarily reflect positions or policies of the American Nurses Association. Furthermore, the information in this book should not be construed as legal or other professional advice.

Published by Nursesbooks.org
The Publishing Program of ANA

American Nurses Association
8515 Georgia Avenue, Suite 400
Silver Spring, MD 20910-3492
1-800-274-4ANA
http://www.Nursesbooks.org/

ANA is the only full-service professional organization representing the nation's 2.9 million Registered Nurses through its 54 constituent member associations. ANA advances the nursing profession by fostering high standards of nursing practice, promoting the economic and general welfare of nurses in the workplace, projecting a positive and realistic view of nursing, and lobbying the Congress and regulatory agencies on healthcare issues affecting nurses and the public.

Page design and composition: Laura C. Johnson, Grammarians, Inc.
Cover design: Stacy Maguire, EyeDea Advertising & Design, Sterling, VA
Production editing: Eric Wurzbacher, ANA • *Copyediting:* Kathy Kelly, Grammarians, Inc.
Proofreading: Gina Wiatrowski, Grammarians, Inc.
Printing: McArdle Printing, Inc., Upper Marlboro, MD

ISBN-13: 978-1-55810-264-4 SAN: 851-3481 2.5M 01/09
First printing January 2009.

Contents

About the Editors

Nancy Dunton, PhD
Director, National Database of Nursing Quality Indicators
Research Associate Professor
University of Kansas School of Nursing

Nancy Dunton is a multi-talented researcher who brings many abilities to the National Database of Nursing Quality Indicators (NDNQI). She has been the director of NDNQI since its inception in 1998, guiding its growth development over the last ten years. Dr. Dunton has made numerous presentations on NDNQI to nurses across the United States and internationally. She has more than 25 years of experience in helping organizations use outcome indicators in decision-making. Dr. Dunton is a Research Associate Professor in the University of Kansas Medical Center's School of Nursing, with a joint appointment in the Department of Health Policy and Management. She has been the principal investigator on more than 20 health and social services research projects and has served on committees for the National Quality Forum, the Agency for Healthcare Quality and Research, and the Committee on National Statistics of the National Academy of Sciences. Dr. Dunton received her PhD in Sociology from the University of Wisconsin–Madison.

Isis Montalvo, RN, MS, MBA
Assistant Director, Nursing Practice & Policy
American Nurses Association

Isis Montalvo is primarily responsible for providing oversight to the National Database of Nursing Quality Indicators® in which 1,400 hospitals currently participate (www.nursingquality.org). Ms. Montalvo has over 20 years of experience in multiple areas of clinical and administrative practice with a focus in critical care and performance improvement. As a former NDNQI Site Coordinator, Quality Specialist, and Nursing Research Chair at a large urban facility, she brings expertise in data analysis, performance improvement, and nursing care evaluation. In 1996, she received her Master's in Business Administration from the University of Baltimore in Maryland and her Master's of Science in Nursing Administration from the University of Maryland. She is a Critical Care Registered Nurse (CCRN) and a member of the American Association of Critical Care Nurses, the American Society of Association Executives/The Center for Association Leadership, the National Association for Healthcare Quality, the American Nurses Association, and Phi Kappa Phi and Sigma Theta Tau Honor Societies.

Acknowledgments

The editors would like to thank the staff nurses who make the daily difference in patient outcomes; the authors for their generosity in sharing their experiences so that others might benefit; the NDNQI project staff who identified hospitals with sustained improvement, checked data for accuracy, and assisted with proofing the manuscripts; Kevin D. Frick, PhD, for his insightful Afterword; Mary Jean Schumann, RN, MSN, MBA, CPNP; and the staff of Nursesbooks.org, the Publishing Program of ANA.

Introduction:
Achieving Sustained Improvements in the Nursing Work Environment, Nursing Workforce Characteristics, and Patient Outcomes

Overview of NDNQI

The National Database of Nursing Quality Indicators® (NDNQI) was established by the American Nurses Association (ANA) in 1998 and has been in operation for 10 years. NDNQI is a program of ANA's National Center for Nursing Quality (NCNQ). ANA's NCNQ encompasses various nursing quality activities that identify and promote nurses' roles in quality. NDNQI is managed by the University of Kansas School of Nursing, under contract to ANA.

NDNQI first issued reports in the third quarter of 1999 with data from fewer than 40 hospitals. As this is written, nearly 1,400 hospitals receive reports (Figure 1).

NDNQI participating hospitals are located in every state, the District of Columbia, and six countries outside of the United States. There are hospitals with fewer than 25 staffed beds, as well as those with over 1,000 beds. There are academic medical centers and nonteaching hospitals. Most NDNQI participants are general acute care hospitals, although specialty hospitals participate as well. Most NDNQI participants are not-for-profits, although for-profit and government hospitals also participate. Many Magnet™ facilities participate, but there are more participants without Magnet recognition. In short, NDNQI participants cover the wide spectrum of hospital types.

Hospitals join NDNQI because they are interested in quality improvement and want data to support

FIGURE 1.
Growth in NDNQI Participation

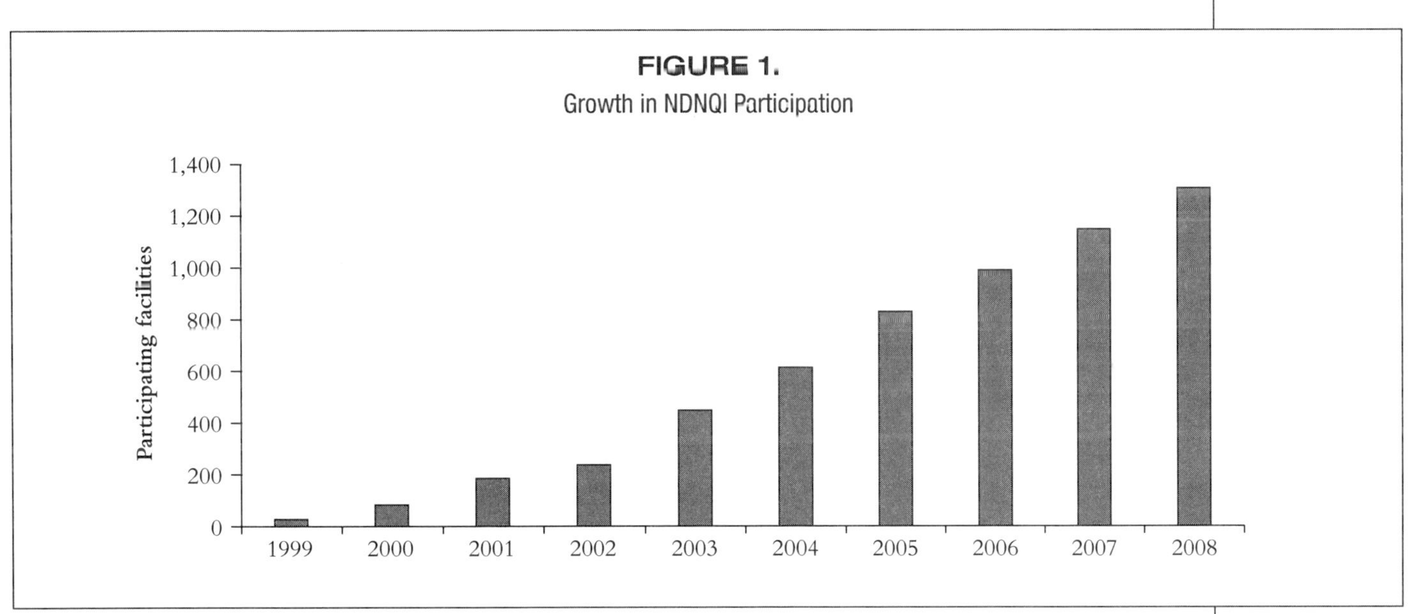

TABLE 1.
NDNQI Hospital Characteristics Compared with Community Hospitals from the American Hospital Association Annual Survey

	NDNQI (%)	AHA (%)
Community Hospitals	97	78
Bed Size		
< 100 Beds	17	49
500+ Beds	12	5
Community Hospital Ownership		
Not-for-Profit	89	58
For-Profit	5	18
Government	6	23
Magnet Recognition, All Hospitals	22	5

Source: 2008 data from the National Database of Nursing Quality Indicators and data from the 2007 Annual Survey by the American Hospital Association.

nursing administration activities. Participants also have the staff and information resources to gather and use data on nursing quality and the nursing work environment. Thus, NDNQI facilities are not representative of all hospitals in the United States (Table 1). Compared with all community hospitals in the American Hospital Association (AHA) annual survey, on average, NDNQI hospitals are larger, more likely to be academic medical centers, have Magnet recognition, and have not-for-profit ownership.

NDNQI has two primary data collection activities: quarterly data on nursing indicators and annual data from the RN surveys of job satisfaction and the nursing work environment. NDNQI's nursing quality indicators include most of the national nursing consensus measures identified by the National Quality Forum (NQF), as well as indicators developed by NDNQI. Appendix A presents a list of the NQF Nursing Consensus measures and Appendix B provides a list of NDNQI indicators and data elements.

The NDNQI began collecting RN Survey data in 2001 with 64 participating hospitals. In 2008, survey data were collected in nearly 700 hospitals, with nearly a quarter-million RN respondents (Figure 2), making it the largest survey of registered nurses in the United States. The survey collects not only information on job satisfaction and the nursing work environment, but also data on contextual items and RN characteristics.

National Trends in Quality Improvement

Concerns over rising healthcare costs and patient safety have resulted in growing public pressure for healthcare reform and provider accountability (Kohn, Corrigan, & Donaldson, 2000). The responses to these pressures have included public reporting, financial incentives for high-quality care, and financial penalties for substandard care. The Centers for Medicare and Medicaid Services (CMS) publish data on healthcare quality measures for hospitals across the United States. A growing number of states require, or are considering requiring, public reporting. Increasingly, nursing quality indicators are among the data being reported. In 2007, the Robert Wood Johnson Foundation provided support for a test of the 15 NQF nursing consensus measures, carried out by the Joint Commission, to determine if they could be reliably collected as a bundle of measures. The report of that study will be published in 2009.

As of October 2008, CMS will no longer reimburse hospitals for the treatment of a number of avoidable adverse events. CMS's goal is to make hospital stays safer for patients by holding the hospital accountable for ensuring they take proper precautions to prevent some reasonably avoidable adverse hospital acquired conditions (CMS 2008). Some of the avoidable events include performing surgery on the wrong body part, hospital acquired infections, or advanced pressure ulcers. Nursing has a role in the prevention of at least four of these conditions (Table 2) and may have a role in others. CMS is also considering eliminating reimbursement for additional avoidable conditions in future years.

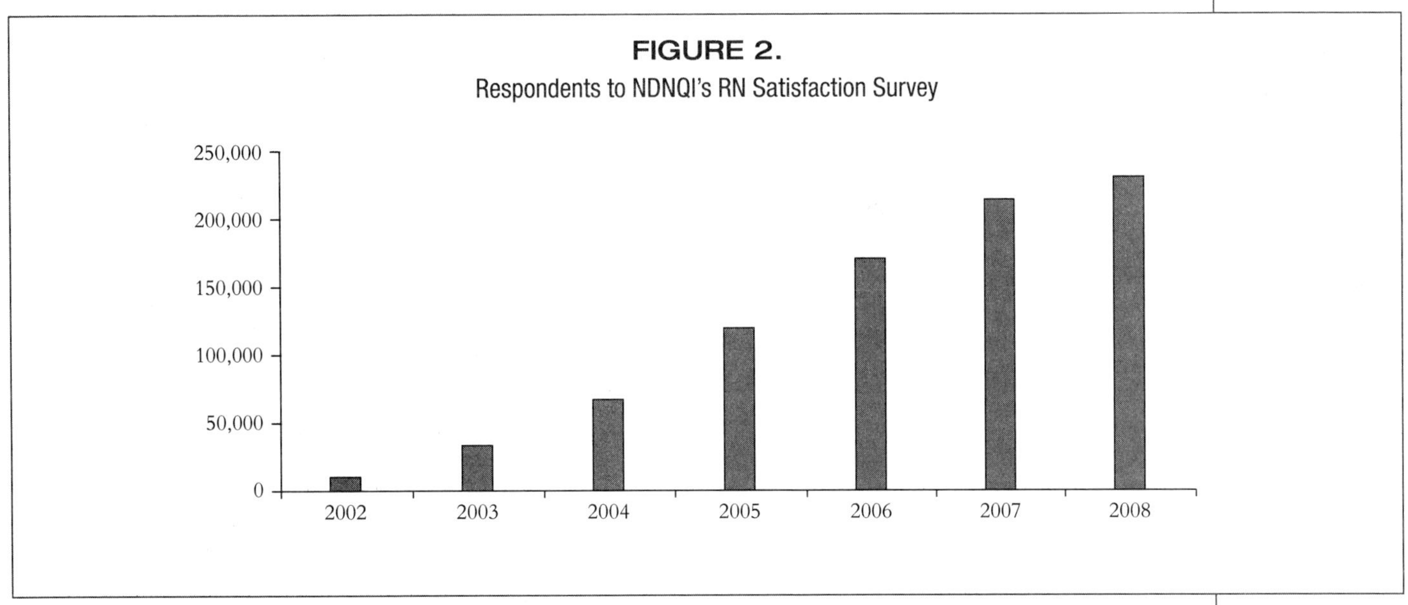

Nursing leaders in hospitals across the nation are monitoring nursing quality measures and searching for successful quality improvement initiatives. NDNQI researchers and other researchers have been successful in establishing the linkages between nurse staffing and patient outcomes, and nursing leaders have been able to use NDNQI for quality improvement. However, staffing is but one consideration in the work environment. Organizational and practice change is difficult to implement and sustain, and is especially difficult if RNs are dissatisfied with their jobs, if there is high RN turnover, and if hospitals are challenged to fill vacant RN positions.

In 2007, ANA published the first monograph presenting the stories of sustained quality improvement in hospitals participating in NDNQI (Montalvo & Dunton, 2007). An overview of quality was provided, and nurses in 14 hospitals described their process and procedures for reducing injury assaults on psychiatric units, reducing patient falls and injury falls, reducing the prevalence of hospital acquired pressure ulcers, improving the completeness of the pain assessment cycle on pediatric units, and improving RN job satisfaction and RN opinions of the nursing work environment.

This volume follows in the footsteps of the initial monograph. Thirteen hospitals describe their processes for achieving sustained improvement in increasing the percentage of RNs with bachelor's degrees in nursing and national specialty certifications, in improving RNs' job satisfaction and retention, and in reducing hospital acquired pressure ulcers and fall rates.

NDNQI identified candidate hospitals through a systematic review of trends in RN survey and quarterly nursing indicator reports. Candidates were asked how they had used their NDNQI reports in achieving success and if they would be interested in publishing their stories. The reader will see in the facility profiles that success stories were found in community hospitals and academic medical centers, in Magnet facilities and non-Magnet facilities, and on a wide variety of unit types. Interestingly, two hospital systems each had two hospitals that had demonstrated this remarkable level of success.

Each of the stories presented in this monograph describes a process of organizational change that was supported and sustained by the hospital leadership but that frequently began with ideas generated by staff nurses in unit councils. Higher levels of communication and team-building were common themes. The

TABLE 2.
CMS Avoidable Adverse Events

Hospital Acquired Conditions

Defined: Reasonably preventable conditions that could be prevented by following evidence-based guidelines, or that are costly or common.

- Foreign object (such as a sponge or needle) inadvertently left in patients after surgery
- Air embolism—an air bubble that enters the bloodstream and can obstruct the flow of blood to the brain and vital organs
- Transfusion with the wrong type of blood
- Severe pressure ulcers*—deterioration of the skin, due to the patient staying in one position too long, that has progressed to the point that tissue under the skin is affected (stage III), or that has become so deep that there is damage to the muscle and bone, and sometimes tendons and joints (stage IV)
- Falls* and trauma:
  - Fracture
  - Joint dislocation
  - Head injury
  - Crushing injury
  - Burn
  - Electric shock
- Catheter-associated urinary tract infection (UTI)*
- Vascular catheter-associated infection*
- Manifestations of poor control of blood sugar levels
- Surgical site infection following coronary artery bypass graft (CABG)
- Surgical site infection following certain orthopedic procedures
- Surgical site infection following bariatric surgery for obesity
- Deep vein thrombosis (a blood clot in a major vein) and pulmonary embolism (blockage in the lungs) following certain orthopedic procedures

Medical Errors That Should Never Happen ("Never Events")

Defined: Events that should never happen in a hospital. If they occur they can cause serious injury or death.

- Surgery on a wrong body part
- Surgery on a wrong patient
- Wrong surgery on a patient

Note: * indicates that nursing has a role in the prevention of these conditions, based on the National Quality Forum Nursing Sensitive Measures.

fall and pressure ulcer prevention stories also are characterized by complex, multifaceted changes in practice. Organizational change is never easy, and these profiles show the level of commitment required for success.

Nursing leaders need models such as these to respond to the public and payer pressures for improved outcomes and to address the effects of the nursing shortage and competition for RNs. Several of the hospitals have provided information on the costs associated with improved outcomes. Importantly, Kevin Frick, PhD, a Johns Hopkins economist, presents an introduction to collecting and using data on costs of organizational change and quality improvement in the Afterword of this monograph. Cost data can be used by nursing leaders to attain support for improvement initiatives.

Recent and Forthcoming NDNQI Developments

NDNQI operates in a continuous state of development and improved services to participating hospitals where nursing occurs. In 2009, advanced reporting and graphics options became available. NDNQI currently provides unit-level indicators where care occurs, and in 2009 NDNQI will undertake a statistical methods development project that will result in the publication of hospital-level indicators. The methods development project also will address the issue of unit-level acuity adjustment, which would enable the inclusion of mixed acuity units in quarterly indicator reporting. Finally, during 2009 and 2010, NDNQI will make existing indicators available on all units for which they are applicable and will undertake the development of new indicators. ANA believes that these advances will aid nursing leaders in their quest for improved patient care and nursing work environments.

As providers of health care, the monograph authors provide exemplars of excellence. The commitment to collecting, reporting, and evaluating unit-level data to assess the quality of nursing care, which provides the framework in which to evaluate nursing practice, with the ultimate goal of improving patient and nursing outcomes. In today's healthcare environment, with its greater focus on quality of care, we applaud the various hospitals profiled for being successful in transforming their units and improving outcomes.

References

Centers for Medicare and Medicaid Services (CMS). (2008). Medicare takes new steps to make your hospital safer. Fact Sheet 8/4/08. Retrieved January 9, 2009, from http://www.cms.hhs.gov/apps/media/press/factsheet.asp?Counter=3227&intNumPerPage=10&checkDate=&checkKey=&srchType=1&numDays=3500&srchOpt=0&srchData=&keywordType=All&chkNewsType=6&intPage=&showAll=&pYear=&year=&desc=false&cboOrder=date

Kohn, L. T., Corrigan, J. M., & Donaldson, M. S. (Eds.). (2000). *To err is human: Building a safer health system.* Committee on Quality of Health Care in America, Institute of Medicine. Washington, DC: National Academy Press.

Montalvo, I. & Dunton, N. (eds.) (2007) *Transforming nursing data into quality care: Profiles of quality improvement in U.S. healthcare facilities.* (American Nurse Association) Nursesbooks.org: Silver Spring, MD.

Education and Certification

Defined:

Highest Nursing Degree:

Determine the highest nursing degree (or U.S. equivalent) for each eligible RN. If an RN has multiple degrees, count only the highest nursing degree. If U.S. equivalent of nursing education obtained in foreign country is uncertain or you don't know their degree, report nursing degree "unknown." Exclude non-nursing degrees.

National Certification:

Certification refers to a tangible recognition of professional achievement in a defined functional or clinical area of nursing. Certification should be counted if it is in a specialty area of nursing practice and granted by a ***national*** nursing organization (for example, ANCC or AACN). Count all nurses who have a nationally recognized certification, even if their area of certification is not the primary specialization on the unit. For example, a nurse who is certified in critical care but works on a medical/surgical unit is to be counted. Nurses with more than one certification should be counted only once, regardless of the number of certifications held.

Exclude:

- Contract/agency staff
- Advanced practice nurses who are not assigned to a single specific unit
- Nurses whose *only* certifications are:
  - Credentialed by an employer in a specialty area or for a clinical procedure
  - For technical skills like ACLS, PALS, or TNCC
  - In an area outside of clinical nursing; for example, case manager

Eligible RNs:

- Count all RN employees (full time, part time, PRN) with direct patient care responsibilities at 50% or greater time who are listed on the staffing roster during the designated period of time
- A nurse who normally works on this unit, but is temporarily absent due to vacation or medical leave should also be counted.

Formulas:

Education:

Number of RNs whose highest level of nursing education is (Nursing Diploma, Associates, Bachelors, Masters, or PhD) divided by the number of RNs on the unit providing direct patient care.

Certification:

Number of RNs with a national specialty certification divided by the number of RNs on the unit providing direct patient care.

Strategies to Support the Advancement of Nursing Educational Levels

Melanie Brewer, DNSc, RN, FNP-BC
Director, Nursing Research
MBrewer@SHC.org

Shirley Righi, MSN, RN, CNEA
Director, Professional Education

Peggy Reiley, PhD, RN
Vice President, Patient Care Services

Scottsdale Healthcare

Editor's Pick

INSIGHTS & IDEAS FROM THIS FACILITY

Hospital investment in education resulted in increasing the proportion of RNs with BSNs and national certifications. One benefit of the program was an increase in RN job satisfaction and a decrease in turnover.

Facility and Unit Summary

Facility	Scottsdale Healthcare (SHC), Shea Campus—Scottsdale, Arizona **www.shc.org**
Facility setting	Full-service hospital serving a large metropolitan area since 1984 • Free-standing outpatient surgery and recovery care center, opened 1982 • Shea Women's Center, opened 2002 • Bariatric Center of Excellence, opened 2005 • Scottsdale Clinical Research Institute and the Virginia G. Piper Cancer Center, offering Phase I and II clinical trials, opened 2005
Teaching status	Teaching hospital
Ownership status	Not-for-profit, three-hospital healthcare system
Community demographics	Scottsdale and Northeastern Maricopa County, Arizona (service area of approximately 185 square miles) • Race/ethnicity: 87% non-Hispanic white and 5% Hispanic • Estimated population 225,000 • 20% of service area population over age 65
Hospital-staffed beds	420 beds, approximately 980 nurses employed
Case mix index	SHC 1.47; Shea campus 1.41
Indicators used	All available NDNQI indicators
System or unit improved	Increase in percentage of bachelor's-prepared nurses on three units at the Shea campus • 3C (Oncology/Hematology)—Increased from 46% to 55% • 5C (Orthopedics)—Increased from 52% to 64% • Neonatal ICU (NICU)—Increased from 50% to 67%
Indicators improved	Certification, education
QI documents used	Nursing quality indicators
NDNQI® participation	Since 2004
Time frame of QI experience	2003–2007

Magnet™ status	Shea campus is one of two Magnet hospitals at SHC
Governance model	17-person board of directors, including one nurse
Awards and recognition	• American Society of Bariatric Surgeons Center of Excellence • Fortune Magazine Best Place to Work—2005, 2006, 2007 • AARP Best Employers for workers over 60—2005 and 2006 • American Heart Association Stroke Center • Thomson Reuters Top Hospitals • Healthgrades Distinguished Hospital Award for Clinical Excellence—2006

UNIT PROFILES

3C

Internal name	3C (Hematology/Oncology)
Size and type	28 beds; med/surg
Staff summary	30 registered nurses (RNs), all chemotherapy certified; 5 licensed practical nurses (LPNs); 10 patient care technicians and nurse's aids
Staff skill mix	60% RNs
Nurse-patient ratio (NHPPD)	1:4
Organizational structure	Nurse manager, Supervisors (charge nurses*), Clinical nurses, Patient-care technicians, Nurse's aids

5C

Internal name	5C (Orthopedics)
Size and type	32 beds; med/surg
Staff summary	45 RNs, 4 LPNs, 32 patient-care technicians and nurse's aids
Staff skill mix	64% RNs; certification 30%
Nurse-patient ratio (NHPPD)	1:5
Organizational structure	Nurse manager, Supervisors (Charge nurses*) Clinical nurses, Patient-care technicians, Nurse's aids

NICU

Internal name	NICU—Level 2
Size and type	20 beds; NICU
Staff summary	49 RNs, 6 patient care technicians, 1 child life coordinator
Staff skill mix	87% RN; certification 54%
Nurse-patient ratio (NHPPD)	1:2
Organizational structure	Nurse manager, Supervisors (Charge nurses*), Clinical nurses, Patient-care technicians (* who support staff in critical thinking and clinical assessment skills)

Strategies to Support the Advancement of Nursing Educational Levels

Melanie Brewer, DNSc, RN, FNP-BC
Director, Nursing Research

Shirley Righi, MSN, RN, CNEA
Director, Professional Education

Peggy Reiley, PhD, RN
Vice President, Patient Care Services

Scottsdale Healthcare

Introductory Summary

Scottsdale Healthcare (SHC) is an independent, not-for-profit health system serving Scottsdale, Arizona, and the surrounding area since 1962. SHC is the city of Scottsdale's largest employer. The organization includes three hospitals: the 337-bed Osborn campus, the 420-bed Shea campus, and the 32-bed Thompson Peak campus that opened in the fall of 2007. The overall percentage of bachelor's-prepared nurses for the system is 45%, and 3.4% are master's prepared. Three units at the Shea campus had notable improvements in the percentage of registered nurses educated at the baccalaureate and master's levels in 2006 through 2007. The three Shea units are described below

Unit 3C is a 28-bed hematology, oncology, and med/surg unit. Chemotherapy certification is required of all RN staff members, and oncology certification (9%) is encouraged. The unit is staffed with 30 RNs, 5 LPNs, and 10 patient care technicians and nurse's aids. Approximately 60% of the total nursing hours are provided by RNs, with 29% provided by unlicensed assistive personnel (UAP) and 5% by LPNs. The nurse-to-patient ratio in 2007 was 1:4. The organizational structure includes a nurse manager, supervisors (charge nurses) who support staff in critical thinking and clinical assessment skills, and bedside nursing staff. Approximately 55% of nurses are prepared at the bachelor's level or higher (18 of 33 nurses with a BSN), and 18% are certified. The case mix index (CMI) for the unit is 1.71.

Unit 5C is a 32-bed orthopedic and med/surg unit with a focus on total joint replacement surgery. The unit is staffed with 45 RNs, 4 LPNs, and 32 patient care technicians and nurse's aids. Approximately 64% of the total nursing hours are provided by RNs, with 29% provided by UAP and 6% by LPNs. Nurse-to-patient ratios in 2007 averaged 1:5. The organizational structure for the unit includes a nurse manager, supervisors, and bedside staff. The percentage of nurses prepared at the bachelor's level or higher is 67% (25 BSN, 1 MSN), and over 30% of the staff are certified. The CMI for the unit is 1.86.

The *Neonatal Intensive Care Unit (NICU)* is a 20-bed designated Level 2 nursery. Infants with gestational age

28 weeks and older are cared for by nurses educated to care for high-risk infants. The unit is staffed with 49 RNs, 6 patient care technicians, and 1 child life care coordinator. Approximately 87% of the total nursing hours are provided by RNs, with the remainder provided by UAP. The percentage of staff nurses prepared at the bachelor's level or higher is 71% (32 BSN, 2 MSN); 54% are certified. Nurse–patient ratios during 2007 were 1:2. The organizational structure for the unit includes a nurse manager, supervisors, and bedside staff. The CMI for the unit is 2.07.

Background

High-quality, safe patient care delivered in the hospital setting has been linked to higher educational levels of registered nurses (Aiken et al., 2003). Increasing the number of RNs prepared at the bachelor's level (BSN) or higher has been shown to decrease the risks of failure to rescue and of mortality for hospitalized patients. Further, Aiken and colleagues found that hospitals with a higher proportion of nurses with a bachelor's degree or higher had decreased surgical mortality rates. In an effort to improve patient outcomes and encourage the use of scientific evidence in nursing practice, SHC initiated a systemwide endeavor to increase the number of hospital RNs prepared at the bachelor's level.

In 2003, senior leadership at SHC increased tuition reimbursement, created a system for loan repayment, and established collaborative relationships with local schools of nursing in order to support RNs who wished to pursue a BSN. Nursing leadership and Human Resources developed a plan to provide education to all interested staff to change the culture of the SHC healthcare system. The journey to Magnet™ had begun, and the impetus to change the system culture to one that strongly supported education across areas moved forward. In addition to senior leadership support for education-related resources, the board of directors was in favor of allocating additional funding for education, given the known benefit of higher RN educational levels to patient outcomes. In addition, increasing support and encouragement to all staff for ongoing education may lead to reduced turnover, higher employee satisfaction, and a greater degree of group cohesion (DiMeglio et al., 2005).

Three clinical units—Oncology/Hematology (3C), Orthopedics (5C), and the Neonatal Intensive Care

FIGURE 1.
Percent of Bachelor's-Prepared RNs

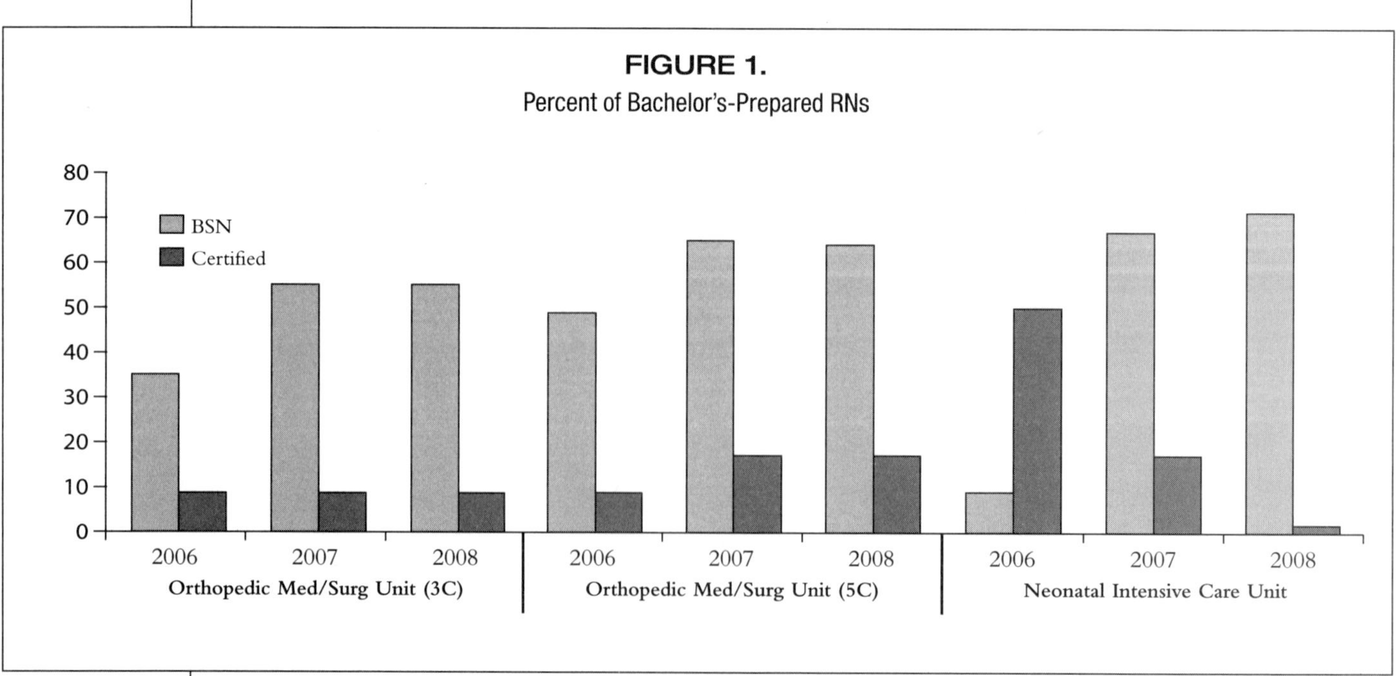

Unit (NICU)—exemplified the benefits of leadership and peer support for advancing the educational level of bedside nurses. Figure 1 illustrates the increase in the percentage of nurses with a BSN who also held a certification from 2006 to 2008. During interviews with staff nurses on each unit, nurses identified several reasons for continuing their education, among them the following:

- The establishment of a learning environment among peers
- Support for educational program participation by the unit manager
- An expectation from leadership that all nurses would continue to grow professionally
- The development of a culture of mentorship and support among nursing colleagues
- Availability of classes on campus and the opportunity to learn with colleagues, which encouraged nurses to participate in both bachelor's and master's programs in nursing

The educational advancement of RNs on these three units was associated with a significant decrease in turnover, improvement in clinical care indicators (including patient falls (Figures 2 and 3), and improvement in patient satisfaction scores (Figure 4).

FIGURE 2.
Improvement in Patient Falls and Falls with Injury (Patient Falls per 1,000 Patient Days—3C)

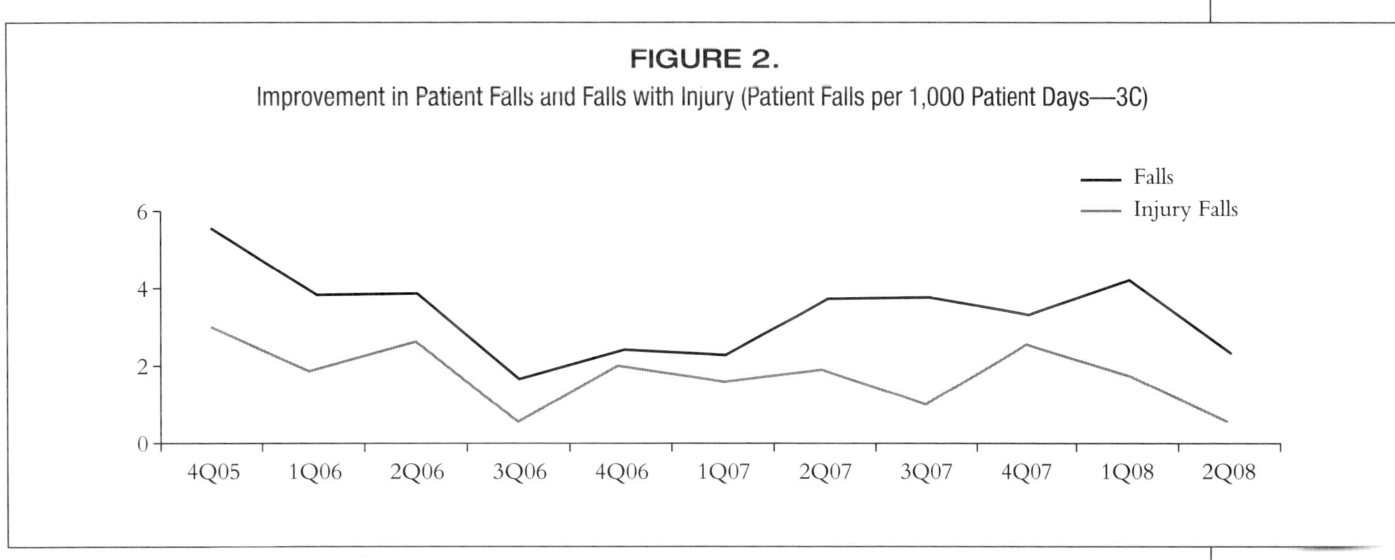

FIGURE 3.
Improvement in Patient Falls and Falls with Injury (Patient Falls per 1,000 Patient Days—5C)

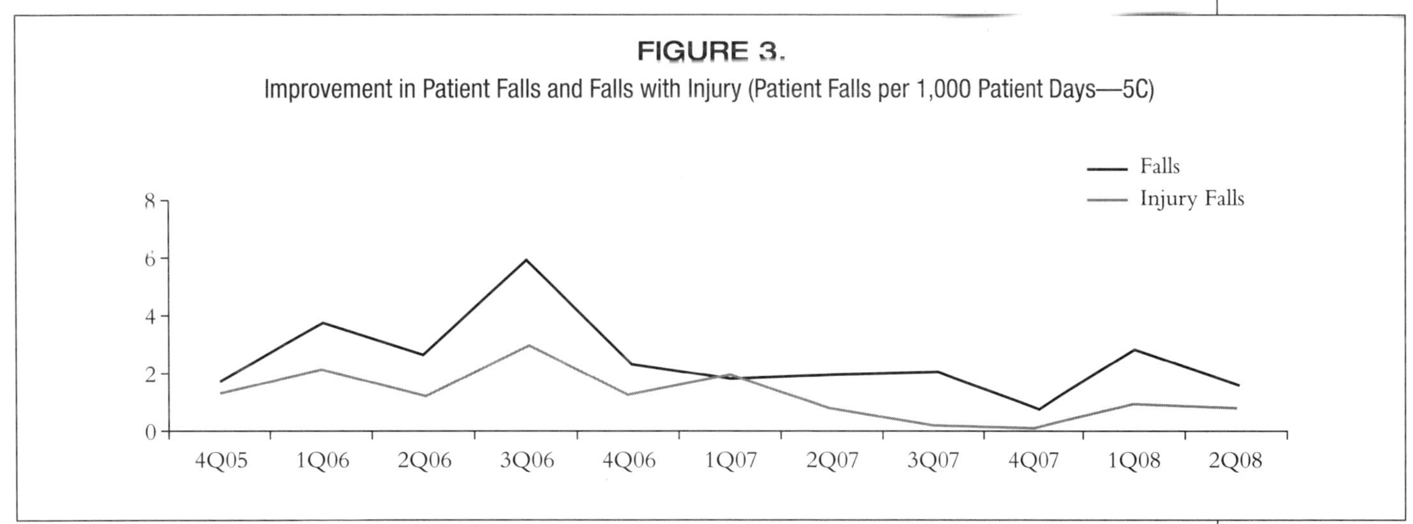

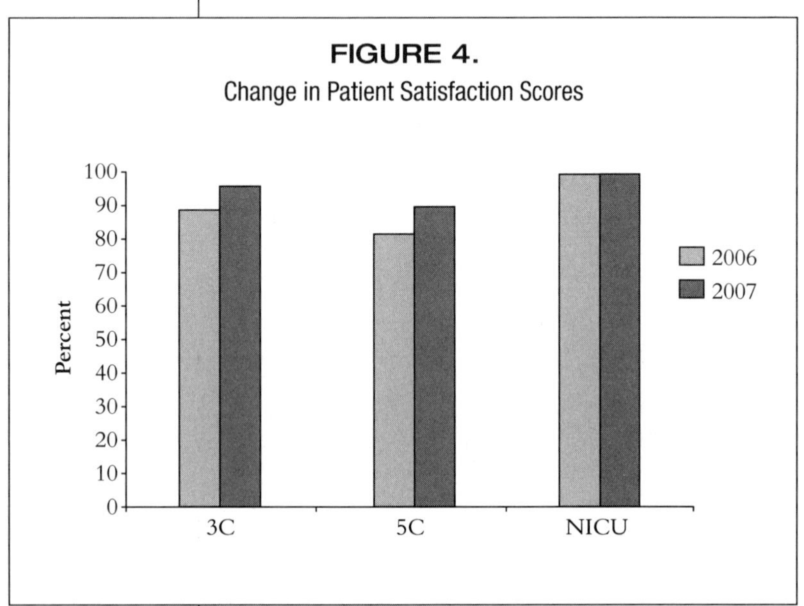

FIGURE 4.
Change in Patient Satisfaction Scores

To improve outcomes of clinical practice, nurses are expected to review and understand their unit's NDNQI scores in order to examine and change practice in response to the findings. The use of evidence in practice at the bedside is strongly supported and is encouraged by nursing leadership, beginning with the chief nurse executive (CNE). Classes are currently under way to educate all RNs in the evidence-based practice process for using findings from scientific literature and internal evidence for clinical decision-making and to inform priorities for conducting research. Nurses who are advancing their education are encouraged to choose projects for school that closely relate to opportunities identified through review of NDNQI benchmarking data.

Organizational Support for Education

In 2003, approximately 73% of nurses in Arizona held an associate's degree in nursing (Randolph, 2007), and SHC was no exception. To increase the number of BSN-prepared nurses, the organization put in place structures and processes to create a culture of professional development for all staff. Nurses were encouraged to further their education through attendance at workshops and conferences, by achievement of certification through professional organizations, or through formal educational programs. A personal development plan, including guidance for development of professional goals, activities to support accomplishment of the goals, and measurement of whether or not the goal was met, is completed by each staff member annually. Nurse managers meet with nurses individually to identify learning needs and goals. Together, they develop a plan of action, which may include returning to school, attending a conference, obtaining professional certification, or pursuing other educational opportunities. Active support of a learning environment at the organizational level generated excitement among nurses as they began to consider new ideas and solutions to problems through education.

The chief nurse executive and the vice president of Human Resources collaborated to develop partnerships with local universities and nursing schools to make classes available on the hospital campus. Two RN-to-BSN programs, two MSN programs, a specialized OR training program, and an LPN-to-RN bridge program were developed and implemented. In addition to providing classrooms and laboratories for instruction, SHC also provides clinical instructors. Assistance is available for education planning, both financially and academically.

Support for education developed at every level of the organization. Many managers, supervisors, and staff nurses are now adjunct faculty and mentor their peers. This collaboration came about because of the strong collaborative relationships with schools of nursing developed through on-site education. Flexible work scheduling is offered to accommodate classes. Managers facilitated scheduling through creative processes such as the use of per diem staff, self-scheduling, and working directly with staff to accommodate their needs. Nurses began to integrate work on clinical problems with school projects. Many of the projects have been implemented in clinical practice, enhancing perceived benefits and communication by staff. As the nurses study and learn together, strong bonds are established. As the enthusiasm for learning and the school-related teamwork occurred, other nurses felt supported to return to school. As the first cohorts of nurses finished their degrees, they began to share with each other that "it wasn't so hard" and encouraged others to attend. Experienced associate's-level nurses and LPNs pursued BSNs. In addition, nurse's aids and health unit coordinators were encouraged and supported by staff nurses and their managers to pursue professional nursing careers.

Cost of Education

Nurses are eligible for tuition reimbursement after 90 days of employment at Scottsdale Healthcare for those who work a minimum of 16 hours per week, and no service commitment is required after the degree is completed. Tuition assistance is provided up-front, removing a significant financial barrier to pursuing further education. As a result, a steady increase has been seen both in tuition reimbursement dollars spent and in the number of participants in the program.

Tuition assistance is available in the amount of $5,250 per year for staff and $6,500 for managers. In 2005, 376 employees participated in a basic RN educational program at a cost of $502,941. For the RN-to-BSN program, 148 nurses participated at a cost of $385,000, and 82 nurses participated in a master's program at a cost of $243,000. Thus, in 2005, SHC spent $1,130,941 on tuition for nurses. The number of participants has increased each year, and 934 nurses are expected to participate in 2008. Figures 5 and 6 illustrate the increasing numbers of participants in the nursing educational advancement programs and include the financial commitment for 2006 and 2007, with projections for 2008. Since the inception of the program, the total tuition cost is estimated to be $6,929,994. Annual tuition cost is approximately $2,309,998. Additional costs include providing the programs on campus, including faculty instructional costs ($72,000 yearly) and remodeling of laboratory space, updating of equipment, and other related costs ($135,000).

FIGURE 5.
RN Educational Program Participants
(Number of Participants in Tuition Assistance Program)

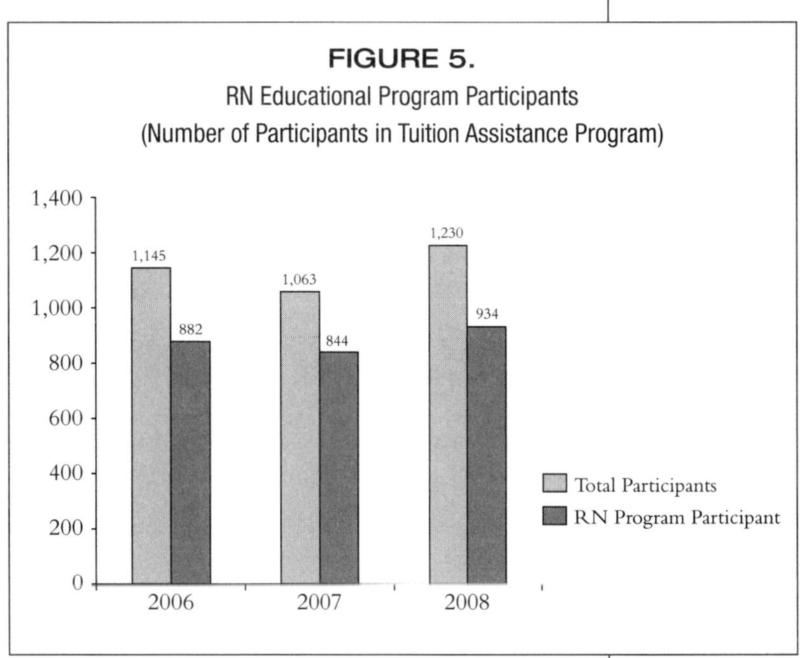

FIGURE 6.
Tuition Assistance Program at SHC
(Dollars Spent on Tuition Assistance)

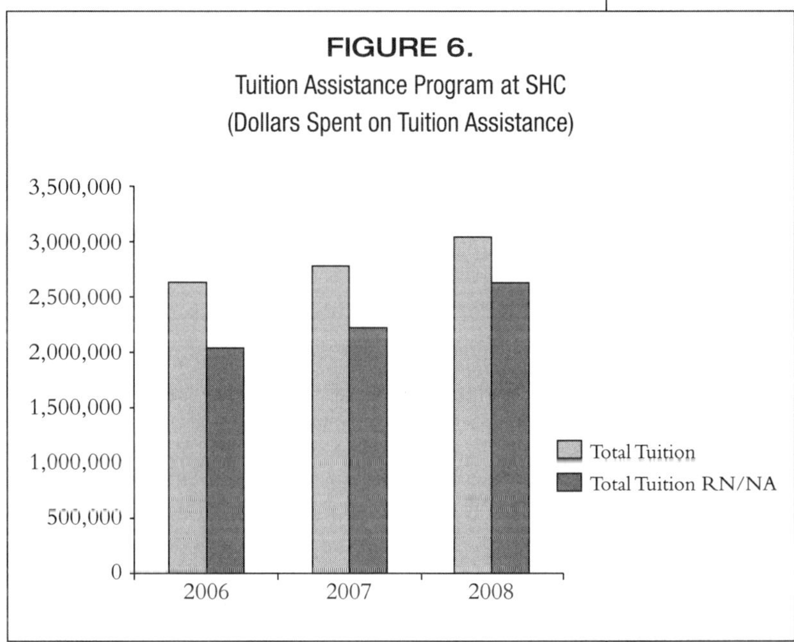

Loan Assistance and Work Study

In 2003, a Nursing Loan Assistance Program (NLAP) was created for direct care nurses, including nursing supervisors and nurse practitioners. The NLAP repays principal and interest on government and commercial loans obtained for undergraduate or graduate nursing education. In addition to the NLAP, a work study program is available. Employees in entry-level positions are paired with mentors who support and guide them in reaching educational goals in nursing. Further, the work study program provides the opportunity to gain experience working with patients and is an effective recruitment tool to retain students upon graduation.

Support for Conference Attendance

Support is available for direct care nurses to attend local, state, and national conferences. Registration and travel costs are often paid for in full. Scottsdale Healthcare Foundation also provides funds for educational conference attendance, with approximately $721,000 in additional funding for nursing staff education. The foundation is a separate nonprofit fund-raising entity. The majority of gifts are from community philanthropists and grateful patients and families. Funds are available by application through a scholarship committee chaired by direct care nurses. Funds are also available for conference attendance as part of the Scottsdale Healthcare Investment in Nursing (SHINE) program, a nursing recognition program. As part of their professional development award, nurses are eligible for funds to support professional organization dues, books and subscriptions, and/or conference attendance. Of the total dollars spent, more than $410,000 was provided to support nurse participation in various conferences and meetings in 2006. The figure for 2007 was slightly increased and is estimated to be $460,000.

Impacts of Education: Staff Outcomes

Increasing the percentage of bachelor's-prepared nurses at SHC Shea has improved patient care outcomes, reduced staff turnover (0% in the NICU in 2007), and generally improved RN satisfaction. As the numbers of BSNs increase, nurses on the units identify a higher level of professionalism, peer-to-peer collaboration, mentorship and support for each other, and commitment to improving outcomes of patient care as part of specific areas of change. Using the NDNQI as a benchmark to evaluate change in nursing practice, improvement was also noted in clinical outcome measures for patients, such as falls with injury (see Figures 2 and 3 on page 9).

Nurses on each of the three units were interviewed to determine the impact of this change on their unit. Several key concepts were identified by the nurses across all three units. Specifically, nurses mentioned mentorship, leadership support, group cohesion and support, the opportunity to work in a learning environment focused on improving outcomes for patients, opportunities to attend educational conferences, and financial support as significant contributors to their successful completion of a bachelor's or master's program.

Mentorship from nurse managers and other nursing leaders in the organization was discussed as a catalyst for consideration of nurses on all three units. Nurses identified the opportunity to attend a national conference, combined with specific guidance from a mentor as to which lectures might be of most benefit, as a significant contributor to the decision to return to school. One nurse mentioned the opportunity to attend a Magnet conference with the director of professional education as being a turning point for her. "She asked me to attend the conference and was enthusiastic about participating in learning opportunities. She encouraged me to go back to school and supported me through the application process."

The role of the nurse manager was identified as a crucial resource to developing and encouraging a learning environment on the clinical unit. The nurse manager provides support for the use of scientific information, and presents a constant challenge to learn more about clinical practice issues and to pursue professional development opportunities.

The NICU manager has observed that nurses recently hired in the NICU already have a bachelor's degree and are interested in neonatal nursing because of the opportunities for ongoing education. Numerous classes are offered each year to enhance clinical knowledge and advance nursing skills. Opportunities to collaborate with advanced practice nurses on improving outcomes for patients contribute to the overall experience of nurses in the NICU. Turnover has dropped to zero in the past year (2007).

Nurses on 3C Unit described the importance of encouragement and mentorship by the nurse manager, the clinical nurse specialist, and nursing colleagues on the unit for making the decision to return to school. The nurse manager continues to mentor nurses to consider returning to school, obtain certification, participate in oncology-related professional organizations, and find other opportunities to advance professionally. Currently, eight nurses are enrolled in a BSN program, two are in a master's program, and six are preparing for the oncology certification exam. The clinical nurse specialist's role in discussing relevant clinical issues that incorporate the timely use of sound evidence for patient care was identified as key to building confidence for entry into a BSN program. In addition, staff nurses who participated in educational programs developed presentations on clinical topics of interest for bedside care and presented these to other staff nurses, further encouraging others to engage in educational activities.

The nurses identified as important elements an environment of open communication among peers to discuss clinical issues and support to each other for problem-solving of patient care concerns. An unintended but significant outcome was the group cohesion that developed as a result of going to school together, resulting in improved working relationships and collegiality. Several nurses have returned to school together for a master's degree. Nurses support and encourage each other to continue their education; in addition, they encourage patient care technicians and nurse's aids working on the unit to pursue a degree. The desire to improve outcomes for patients and to provide additional support to families of cancer patients was identified as a strong motivator for continued interest in additional education and shared accountability for practice. Through participation in SHINE, the SHC professional advancement and recognition program, nurses implement evidence in practice and provide leadership to nurses across the organization.

As a result of the increased proportion of BSNs, nurses have become engaged in the process of guiding the direction of unit priorities and lending support to development of new staff. During the past 2 years, the unit culture changed dramatically to one of self-direction and self-governance, and accountability to the group is now the norm. The nurses possess a "can-do" attitude for problem-solving and improving unit outcomes. Turnover has dropped significantly, and nursing satisfaction levels have improved.

Nurses on 5C Unit described the importance of the culture of promoting continued education at SHC as a strong support for returning to school. The nurse manager is currently in a master's program and provides mentorship to staff currently in school or considering an educational program. Recognition of career goals and mentorship is of prime importance. One nurse, who came to the unit as a housekeeper, identified the importance of collaboration and support from her peers in her decision to enter an RN program initially, and now to completing a BSN program. She intends to continue her education to the doctoral level and to continue her work at the bedside. Several nurses mentioned that on-campus nursing leadership courses provided a first step to "try out" a return to school. Once they had completed one or two courses, several nurses returned to school together. Resources available on campus—including library support and education for accessing literature to improve evidence-based care—were identified as important factors in continuing educational pursuits after completion of the BSN program.

Nurses identified a sense of teamwork on the unit as a significant outcome of the higher proportion of BSNs. After completion of a BSN program, several nurses had the confidence to begin and implement a project to improve practice outcomes. Collaboration with physicians is strongly supported by the nurse manager, and problem-solving is an expectation of every nurse. Nurses described the importance of education in providing the tools needed to solve problems and improve communication. Sharing ideas and discussing new strategies with colleagues were identified as a significant change that came with higher levels of education. Patient outcome measures and turnover have improved since 2006.

Recognition of accomplishments related to education has been a priority among nursing leaders at SHC. Nurses who attain certification, a BSN, or an advanced degree, or who participate in the SHINE program, are recognized at luncheons and through a $2-per-hour ($4,160/year) increase in salary. Nurses are continually recognized for their accomplishments and for their contributions to educating colleagues and for improved patient outcomes.

Conclusions and Implications

In general, a higher proportion of RNs educated at the bachelor's level or higher decreases the risks of harm to patients and improves outcomes of care (Aiken et al., 2003). Through an organized effort to increase the number of BSNs at Scottsdale Healthcare Shea and to provide advanced educational opportunities for all nurses, the percentage of nurses with a bachelor's degree or higher has increased. The result: dramatic ongoing improvements in how nurses think about their work and in professional accountability for providing quality nursing care.

As the proportion of BSNs at the bedside has increased, the professional environment for patient care has improved. Communication and collaboration with physicians have improved and led to further improvement in patient and family care, as well as higher levels of unit-related job satisfaction verbalized by both physicians and nurses. In addition, nurses with bachelor's degrees have encouraged clinicians among other disciplines to return to school, and the percentage of professionals with advanced degrees has increased throughout the SHC system.

Several nurses currently are pursuing advanced education through such programs as a master's in healthcare innovation, master's in leadership and education, doctorate of nursing practice, and other doctoral degrees. Through leadership in the Nurse Practitioner Council, the Nursing Research Council, and the Nurse Quality Council, nurses with advanced degrees are improving the SHC healthcare system clinically and organizationally.

References

Aiken, L., Clarke, S., Cheung, R., Sloane, D., & Silber, J. (2003). Educational levels of hospital nurses and surgical patient mortality. *Journal of the American Medical Association, 290,* 1617–1623.

DiMeglio, K., Lucas, S., Padula, C., Piermont, N., Piatek, C., et al (2005). Group cohesion and nurse satisfaction: A team-building approach. *Journal of Nursing Administration, 35*(3), 110–120.

Randolph, P. (2007). Annual Reports from Arizona Nursing Programs. *Arizona Nurses Association.* Retrieved August 10, 2008, from http://www.azbn.gov/documents/education/Annual%20Report%20Analysis%202007.pdf

Promoting Specialty Certifications among Staff Nurses

Debbie Poole, RN, MSN, NEA-BC
Executive Director, Trauma/Postsurgical Services
dkpoole@stmarys.org

Linda Appel, RN, BSN, CMSRN
Staff Development Specialist

Susan Schaefer, RN, BSN, CMSRN
Charge Nurse, General Postsurgical

Mary Moll, RN, MSN, NEA-BC
Executive Director, Medical Services

Sheila Hauck, RN, MSN, NEA-BC
Executive Director, Professional Practice

Rebecca P. Winsett, RN, FNP, PhD
Nurse Scientist

St. Mary's Medical Center

Editor's Pick

INSIGHTS & IDEAS FROM THIS FACILITY

Mentoring and arranging for a local certification test site lead to an increase in the number of RNs with specialty certifications. The multifaceted initiative that began with one unit type is now expanding to others.

Facility and Unit Summary

Facility	St. Mary's Medical Center—Evansville, Indiana **www.stmarys.org**
Facility setting	Areas of specialty include cardiac services; trauma; cancer care; women's health; children's health; and neuroscience, orthopedic, and rehabilitation services. • St. Mary's Rehabilitation Institute is a 35-bed acute rehabilitation facility on the main campus, accredited by the Commission on Accreditation of Rehabilitation Facilities (CARF) • Level II Trauma Center verified by the American College of Surgeons, Committee on Trauma • Cancer Program accredited by the American College of Surgeons Commission on Cancer • Helicopter transport service accredited by the Commission on Accreditation of Transport Services (CAMTS)
Teaching status	Community hospital—nonteaching
Ownership status	Private nonprofit (Ascension Health); the largest Catholic institution and largest nonprofit health system in the United States
Community demographics	• Geographic service area primarily Vanderburgh, Warrick, and Posey counties in southwestern Indiana, with a significant number of patients from bordering western Kentucky and southern Illinois • Evansville is the third largest city in Indiana. It has a metropolitan service area of 300,000 people, with one additional acute care hospital in city. • Approximately 19% of service area population is over age 65
Hospital-staffed beds	299 beds, including newborn nursery
Case mix index (CMI)	1.59
Indicators used	Nursing specialty certifications
System or unit improved	Hospital-wide across multiple specialties; the medical/surgical units as a whole are featured in this article
Indicator improved	Percentage of nurses with specialty certifications
QI documents used	NDNQI % nursing specialty certifications
Time frame of QI experience	2002 to 2007

NDNQI® participation	Since January 2006
Magnet ™ status	Application for Magnet designation made in June 2008
Governance model	Shared governance model consisting of five governing councils: Nursing Alliance Assembly; Clinical Practice; Professional Development and Education; Recruitment, Retention, and Recognition; and Nursing Quality and Research
Awards and recognitions	• American Heart Association, Get with the Guidelines: Coronary Artery Disease Bronze Performance Achievement Award—2008 • Family Friendly Award for Health & Benefit Programs presented by Evansville Chamber of Commerce, Workforce Development, and Evansville Human Resources Association—2007 • *US News & World Report* Get with the Guidelines for achieving 85% compliance in each of the four measures in heart failure for 12 consecutive months—2007 • Ascension Health recognition for zero birth injuries since January 2005—2007 • An American Association for Respiratory Care as a Quality Respiratory Care Institution—2007 • "Best Employer for Workers Over 50" by AARP—2006

UNIT PROFILE

Internal name	Multiple med/surg units
Size and type	2 postsurgical (61 beds), 3 medical (84 beds), and 1 cardiac (48 beds)
Staff summary	2% MSNs, 38% BSNs, 49% ADNs, 11% diplomas. 13% non-nursing BAs/BSs
Staff skill mix	Units average 60% RNs, assisted by patient care technicians and clerical support staff
Nurse-patient ratio (NHPPD)	1:5–6 days, 1:6–8 nights
Organizational structure	CNO/Senior Vice President, Executive director or VP for each service line, Unit director or manager, Unit staff

Promoting Specialty Certifications among Staff Nurses

Debbie Poole, RN, MSN, NEA-BC
Linda Appel, RN, BSN, CMSRN
Susan Schaefer, RN, BSN, CMSRN
Mary Moll, RN, MSN, NEA-BC
Sheila Hauck, RN, MSN, NEA-BC
Rebecca P. Winsett, RN, FNP, PhD

St. Mary's Medical Center

Introductory Summary

An assessment of learning needs at St. Mary's Medical Center (SMMC) identified that promoting certification was a professional goal of the medical/surgical (med/surg) staff. A specific med/surg council created a strategic plan to facilitate the preparation for med/surg certification well before the hospital adopted a formalized Shared Governance council structure, consisting of five governing councils: Nursing Alliance Assembly; Clinical Practice; Professional Development and Education; Recruitment, Retention, and Recognition; and Nursing Quality and Research. The plan led to an increase in the percentage of registered nurses (RNs) with med/surg certifications. Other units and specialties within the hospital later adopted the model created by the med/surg specialty.

Achieving med/surg nursing specialty certification was a goal that emerged from a learning needs assessment performed by the med/surg staff development specialist. In 2001, the med/surg areas became interested in establishing their identity as a unique specialty. A review of Magnet™ organizations indicated that increased specialty certification is a characteristic of nursing excellence. Increasing med/surg certifications was adopted as a goal by the med/surg council, which consisted of representatives of six med/surg units. In 2002, the first year the med/surg plan was implemented, 4 RNs achieved certification. Commitment to the plan increased over the next 4 years, with 27 more RNs certified. As the unit nurses discussed barriers to success, the education council began to implement innovative strategies to entice more nurses to pursue certification and support their efforts toward certification. Strategies that were developed to promote certification included mentoring, role modeling, review classes, fiscal resources, prepayment of certification fees by the institution, on-site testing, and recognition. Over the course of 4 years, med/surg certifications increased, and the experience of the med/surg nurses was used as a process model for other specialty certifications within the hospital.

Promotion of certification became galvanized in the 2007 nursing strategic plan with a goal to increase the number of certified nurses by 4.0% over the FY 2006 level of 17.5%. This was an ambitious goal for a

299-bed acute care community hospital. At the end of 2007, 48% of med/surg nurses were certified, an improvement of 30 percentage points. This compared favorably with the National Database of Nursing Quality Indicators (NDNQI®) peer group mean of 9%. Further, improvements were also seen in the three critical care units, where 36% of SMMC nurses were certified as compared with the NDNQI peer group mean of 13%. In addition to the med/surg and intensive care units, 66% of nursing directors and 100% of the senior nursing leadership have achieved specialty certification. As the retention rate for certified nurses remains high, pursuing certification has become a distinctive mark for nursing excellence.

Background

Specialty certification is defined by the American Board of Nursing Specialties (ABNS) as "the formal recognition of the specialized knowledge, skills, and experience demonstrated by the achievement of standards identified by a nursing specialty to promote optimal health outcomes" (ABNS, 2007). A study of 11,427 nurses identified values and challenges to specialty certification (ABNS, 2006). Certification was found to be a valuable method for nurses to differentiate themselves in the workplace, enhance personal and professional satisfaction, and validate specialized knowledge. Challenges to certification included poor institutional support and costs. As a result of this survey, the ABNS has encouraged hospital efforts to promote certification. Several benefits of certification have been presented in nursing literature, including the validation of expert knowledge, increased professional credibility, sense of personal accomplishment and personal satisfaction, professional challenge and commitment, and an indicator of personal growth (Cliff & Martinez, 2004; Stromberg et al., 2005; Weeks, Ross, & Roberts, 2006). These values are critical to a culture of nursing excellence and are recognized as key indicators of Magnet-designated facilities by the American Nurses Credentialing Center.

In the learning needs assessment performed in early 2002, specialty certification surfaced as a need for the same reasons as identified by the ABNS. The Med/Surg Education Council had a desire to establish and recognize med/surg as a specialty. The council noted that certified nurses in other specialties received tangible recognition, with plaques and pictures displayed on the unit, and decided strategies for recognition needed to be included in the development plan. The council set goals to (1) develop a plan to increase med/surg certifications, which would lead to recognition of med/surg as a unique and recognized specialty, (2) improve the image of med/surg nursing in the hospital and among med/surg nurses, and (3) create a strategic plan that included having more RNs certified in med/surg. The council also evaluated local education classes and regional conferences, along with the competencies assessed during RN orientation, and felt that specialty certification would increase competency among staff RNs. To increase interest in med/surg certification, membership in the specialty's professional organization, the Academy of Medical–Surgical Nurses, was encouraged.

Strategies Used

The strategies used to promote specialty certification came from the initial efforts of the Med/Surg Education Council, including formal review sessions that were held in advance of a med/surg certification review conference, the review conference itself, informal interactive review sessions, classes with test-taking skill reviews, and collaboration with another hospital to obtain a local testing site. These strategies were supported through both fee reimbursement and recognition of certification through the Career Advancement Program. The other nursing units have used the med/surg model for promoting certification within their nursing specialty, with increases in certifications seen in both critical care, step-down, and pediatric units.

Formal Review Sessions

The Med/Surg Education Council developed a certification review course based upon the certification preparation exam questions and core curriculum review areas. The course was initially set up in eight weekly sessions between June and September to coincide with the fall testing dates. Review sessions were held at the hospital, with meals provided to the participants. Internal experts were used as presenters. The review sessions were open to all interested nurses regardless of intent to test for certification. Sixty RNs attended at least one session, with an average of 35 RNs attending each of the review sessions. This included nurses from other specialty areas who wanted to increase their knowledge in the content areas.

Medical–Surgical Review Conference

In addition to the weekly review sessions, the council developed a two-day med/surg nursing review conference based on the med/surg core curriculum review material and invited the Academy of med-surg Nursing (AMSN) director of education to speak. This conference was held at the hospital just prior to the fall testing date. Nurses on the postsurgical units who were willing to test for certification were allowed to attend the AMSN national conference if they were willing to test for certification while attending the conference. Four RNs who participated in the review sessions were certified in the fall of 2002. Three achieved certification as Certified Medical Surgical Registered Nurses and one was Orthopedic Nurse Certified. They were recognized in the hospital newsletter and on unit display boards.

Informal Interactive Review Sessions

The Med/Surg Education Council was somewhat disappointed with the low number of RNs testing for certification after the initial plan rollout, so in late 2003, currently certified med/surg nurses (n = 10) were surveyed regarding reasons to certify and the best approaches for preparation. The responses identified pride and personal satisfaction as the primary reasons to certify. Approaches to study included more interactive review sessions, with emphasis on test-taking, and not having to travel away from home to take the certification exam. Fear of failure was also a barrier to willingness to test, and some staff chose to test anonymously. Pay was not identified as a reason to pursue certification by any of the respondents.

Based upon the feedback from the certified nurses, the council decided to provide additional educational offerings to prepare for certification. Small group study sessions were planned as well as a short lecture series. An all-day review course was provided with review materials on CDs. Core curriculum review CDs were purchased for each of the six med/surg units represented on the council. At the suggestion of the certified nurses, interactive sessions were provided in the evening. The sessions remained open to any interested staff, as the review sessions were instrumental in developing knowledge base and critical thinking skills, even if some staff did not intend to seek certification. Again, the AMSN director of education was engaged to provide a 2-day med/surg certification review course. Nursing leadership also sought out other educational and professional meetings that would be of benefit and encouraged RNs to attend.

Test-Taking Skills

Test-taking skills were identified as a barrier for some nurses who had not engaged in formal education for a number of years. As age of the RN staff appeared to be a factor in choosing to seek certification, there was a focus to target younger RNs in order to energize the initiative. The nursing director of the postsurgical unit and the staff development specialist for med/surg prepared for the certification exam along with the staff in order to provide role models and increase interest among the older RNs. It was also felt that the interactive sessions using preparation questions along with discussing the critical thinking rationale would help allay test-taking anxiety and enhance test-taking skills.

Collaborative Local Testing Site

In evaluating the possible reasons for the low number of participants testing for certification after the sessions, it was identified that it would be helpful to provide a local testing site. SMMC collaborated with a neighboring hospital to garner enough interest and participation to offer a test site locally. Subsequently, the number of RNs taking the exam increased to around 10 new certifications in FY 2007. That trend is continuing with 10 new certifications in the first 6 months of FY 2008.

Fee Reimbursement

To ensure that there was not a financial barrier to testing, funding was procured to help offset the cost of the certification exam. The hospital's foundation and supportive physicians contributed funding to offset the initial costs of the educational offerings. Monies were used to pay for travel to conferences and to prepay certification testing fees on a conditional basis. If candidates did not test or were unsuccessful, they agreed to reimburse the testing fee. Each on-site medical–surgical review course costs approximately $5,000. The costs for initial certification exams and renewals for med/surg certification have been approximately $3,500 annually. SMMC invested approximately $1,200 to purchase core curriculum review CDs for the seven med/surg units. Participants were paid their hourly base rate to attend the 2-day med/surg certification review course and the on-site core curriculum review sessions. The cost of staff time, nearly $21,000, has been the greatest expense associated with the promotion of certifications and clearly demonstrated to staff RNs that there was institutional support for certification. Thus, annually, SMMC has invested nearly $30,000 in promoting certifications among med/surg RNs, or approximately $600 per certified med/surg RN (n = 48 in FY 2007). When other specialties are included, the organizational investment for certification and recertification testing fees alone increases to $15,000 annually.

Recognition of Certification in the Career Advancement Program

In 2007, a Career Advancement Program (CAP) was put into place that provided additional opportunities for certification recognition. To be recognized at the highest level of the CAP, an RN must achieve and sustain certification. There is financial recognition for each CAP level, with a potential for a $4,000 bonus for the highest level. The CAP application must be renewed annually.

Use of the Med–Surg Model

Because of the interest from other specialty units, staff development specialists began hosting informational sessions for all specialties on the certification process and benefits. These sessions generated interest from orthopedics, progressive care, oncology, renal, vascular access, and case management. Certifications have increased in those areas as well.

Results

Four consequences have been identified with the effort to increase med/surg nursing certifications:

1. The model developed by the med/surg council paved the way for other specialties to organize review courses and increase the number of certified nurses (see Table 1).
2. Turnover rates at SMMC remain much lower than regional and state comparison groups.
3. Patient satisfaction has improved.
4. RN job satisfaction has improved.

From SMMC's initial four certified med/surg RNs in 2002, successive years have shown an increase in med/surg certifications. In 2004, 10 new certifications were achieved, with an additional 10 in 2005, 11 in 2006, and 7 in 2007 (see Figure 1). Feedback from the RNs showed that providing a local testing site was seen as the primary facilitator to promoting certification.

Using the model developed for the med/surg nurses, a review course with a national speaker was arranged on-site for nursing leadership. All eight nursing executive leaders and many of the nursing directors successfully obtained nursing administration certification. Most of the executive directors and directors also held certification in their respective clinical areas.

Although the effort to study for a specialty certification is an individual choice, the strategies employed at SMMC have been a recipe for success. While nurse retention and nurse and patient satisfaction certainly result from multiple factors, over the past several years there has been an improvement in each of these areas. Of the current 510 RNs eligible for certification, 185 (36%) are certified in 34 specialties. In addition, 19 RNs hold certifications in more than one specialty. Therefore, certification has become an expression of nurses becoming involved in nursing excellence at SMMC. Professional development endeavors may be a factor in the low turnover rates experienced at SMMC, which has a nurse turnover rate of 2.72%, compared with a regional rate of 6.29% and a state rate of 3.53% (IHHA, 2008).

Another measure of success, which may be attributed in part to the increasing number of certifications, is patient satisfaction (Cary, 2001). In November 2006, SMMC implemented a new care-delivery model, with relationship-based care (RBC) (Koloroutis, 2004). Professional nursing is one of the seven RBC model components. Over 700 nurses attended an education program on RBC, which discussed professional nursing and the importance of specialty certification. It was during this initiative that the relationship-based care behaviors were integrated as a part of patient-centered care. Inpatient satisfaction with SMMC was at a record high in 2007, with a percentile ranking in the upper 90s. In 2008, the overall inpatient satisfaction raw mean score was significantly higher than the national mean for comparable facilities (8.90 vs. 8.09; $p < .05$), ranking in the 99th percentile.

Nursing-specific satisfaction surveys were not administered at SMMC prior to 2006, so the degree of improvement for the professional status of nursing and the professional development scores from the initial promotion of specialty certifications cannot be determined. The professional status of nursing t-scores on the NDNQI-Adapted Index of Work Satisfaction

TABLE 1.
SMC Organizational Improvements in RN Certifications by Unit (percent)

Specialty	Baseline % RNs with National Certification	FY07 % RNs with National Certification	Percent Point Change
Med/Surg	3.2	43.6	40.0
Adult Critical Care	12.0	45.5	34.0
NICU	5.3	11.5	6.0
IP Rehab	22.7	45.5	23.0
Mental Health	50.0	64.7	15.0

FIGURE 1.
Med/Surg Certifications at SMMC

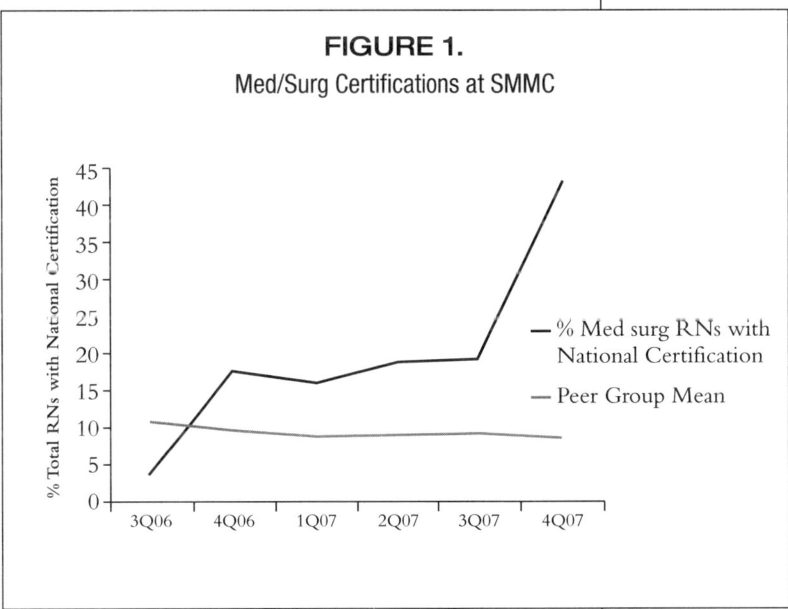

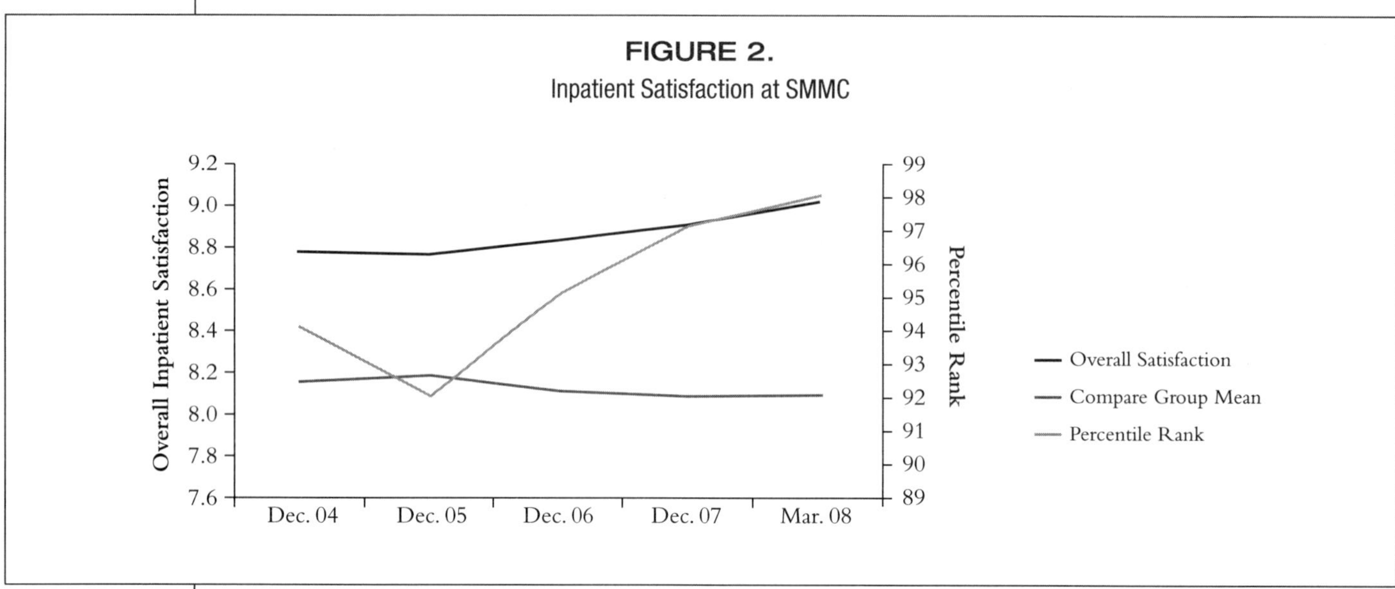

FIGURE 2.
Inpatient Satisfaction at SMMC

improved from 60.97 in 2006 to 62.60 in 2007, both of which are in the high satisfaction range. The professional development t-scores on the NDNQI-Adapted Nursing Work Index improved from the moderate satisfaction rating of 58.48 in 2006 to a high satisfaction rating of 60.34 in 2007.

The CAP has evolved into a meaningful mark of nursing excellence, with a significant number of staff nurses participating annually. The program requires points to be acquired through participation in four professional practice areas, as outlined in Table 2.

Nurses' levels of achievement are formally indicated as the following: Level II for those nurses actively developing their professional practice, Level III for those nurses who demonstrate a well-developed professional practice and serve as resources for colleagues, and Level IV for those nurses who demonstrate expertise in professional practice and serve as role models for colleagues. In the first year of CAP, 55 RNs participated, with 17 achieving Level II, 21 achieving Level III, and 17 achieving Level IV. In the first of two 2008 opportunities to participate, there were 22 repeat participants and 16 new participants, with 3 achieving Level II, 27 achieving Level III, and 8 achieving Level IV. Certification became a requirement to achieve Level IV in the second 2007 offering. Several participants plan to obtain certification to attain Level IV. The success of the program is viewed as indicating increased interest in advancing both professional development and certification.

The value placed on certification has recently spread to the pediatrics unit, which had only 3 out of 23 RNs certified. Twelve additional RNs recently achieved pediatric certification. Currently, 62% of the eligible pediatric RNs are certified.

Conclusions and Implications

As the journey to nursing excellence has spread throughout the organization, a heightened interest in advancing nursing practice is apparent. Certification has become a mark of nursing excellence at SMMC, fostering a sense of pride and personal accomplishment. Several strategic initiatives are thought to have had a major impact on the growth in certifications.

Interest in certification increased among registered nurses when the review sessions were tailored for the target audience. Providing the review materials through multiple venues made the older RNs feel more comfortable with the content and with their test-taking skills. The review courses and informational

TABLE 2.
Career Advancement Program (CAP) Criteria

CAP Criteria Category	Level II Points Required	Level III Points Required	Level IV Points Required*
Enrichment and Professional Development	5	8	11
Performance Improvement and Innovation	5	8	11
Leadership and Collegiality	3	6	11
Collaborative Practice and Community	3	6	11
Choice Points	4	7	6
Total Points	20	35	50

* Specialty certification & research participation required.

sessions were intentionally planned to help keep those interested on target with the deadlines and to facilitate access to resources and registration materials.

Arranging for a local test site is thought to have had one of the greatest impacts on the number of registered nurses taking the exam. If travel is required to take the certification exam, it continues to be seen as a barrier because of the financial and family burden. Increases in the numbers of staff taking the certification exam were seen when the travel expense associated with distant testing sites was eliminated. Increases were also seen in the numbers of staff taking the certification exam when arrangements were made for conditional prepayment of exam fees. To date, all requests for payment of certification fees have been honored. The elimination of the financial barriers resulted in an increased interest in taking the certification exam.

Role modeling has become one of SMMC's strategic initiatives in advancing professionalism among nurse leaders and staff. Momentum was gained as staff saw success in others. Those who lacked confidence or had a fear of failing were encouraged and supported by those who had been through the process. Promoting a culture of safe risk-taking was a component of overcoming the fear of failure. The staff became more comfortable with the certification process after seeing older leaders successfully complete the process. As new generations continue to enter the nursing workforce, it will be important to continue entertaining new strategies to engage multiple generations.

Although the journey started in 2002, the early initiatives have led to a high percentage of certified nursing staff in 2007. Specialty certification has certainly had an impact on the work environment and on SMMC's nursing staff. The successes described support the evidence of the value of certification and the positive outcomes associated with certification. Med/surg has become recognized and valued as a specialty within itself, and the staff have a sense of pride and accomplishment. This has translated to patients through the delivery of an exceptional patient experience by expert nurses.

References

American Board of Nursing Specialties (ABNS). (2006). *Values of specialty nursing certification survey: Executive summary.* Retrieved August 4, 2008, from http://www.nursingcertification.org/pdf/executivesummary

American Board of Nursing Specialties (ABNS). (2007). *Promoting Excellence in Nursing Certification.* Retrieved August 4, 2008, from http://www.nursingcertification.org

Cary, A. H. (2001). Certified registered nurses: results of the Study of the Certified Workforce. *American Journal of Nursing 2001, 101*(1), 44–52.

Cliff, B., & Martinez, J. (2004). Value of nursing certification [Electronic version]. *Journal of Hospice and Palliative Nursing, 6*(3), 191–192.

Indiana Hospital & Health Association (IHHA). (2008). *HR Benchmarking Survey Report.* Retrieved from IHHA's password protected web site for members only.

Koloroutis, M. (Ed.). (2004). *Relationship-Based Care.* Minneapolis, MN: Creative Health Care Management, Inc.

Stromborg, M., Niebuhr, B., Prevost, S., Fabrey, L., Muenzen, P., Spence, C., et al. (2005). Specialty certification: More than a title. *Nursing Management, 36*(5), 36–46.

Weeks, S., Ross, A., & Roberts, P. (2006). Certification and Magnet hospitals: Will certification advance your career and improve patient outcomes? *American Journal of Nursing, 106*(7), 74–76.

RN Job Satisfaction

The *NDNQI RN Satisfaction Survey* contains the NDNQI® adaptation of Stamps' (1997) *Index of Work Satisfaction* (adapted with permission of Dr. Paula Stamps). Stamps defines job satisfaction as "the extent to which people like their jobs" (p. 13), and "views it as a complex, multidimensional construct that captures individual's reactions to specific components of their work" (Taunton, et al, 2004, p. 102). The *NDNQI-Adapted Index of Work Satisfaction* subscales are defined below:

- *Task:* Activities that must be done as a regular part of the job
- *Nurse–Nurse Interactions:* Formal and informal contact among nurses during working hours
- *Nurse–Physician Interactions:* Formal and informal contact with physicians during working hours
- *Decision-making:* Management policies and practices related to decision-making
- *Autonomy:* Amount of independence, initiative, and freedom permitted or required in daily work activities
- *Professional Status:* Importance or significance of the job, both in nurses' and others' view
- *Pay:* Cash remuneration and fringe benefits received for work performed

Also included are the NDNQI adaptation of selected items of the Aiken and Patrician (2000) Revised Nursing Work Index (adapted with permission of Dr. Linda Aiken). Aiken and Patrician developed this instrument as an organizational environment measure. The NDNQI-Adapted Nursing Work Index subscales are defined below:

- *Professional Development:* Opportunity and access to career development
- *Supportive Nursing Management:* Satisfaction with unit managers in relation to decision, support, and consultation
- *Nursing Administration:* The visibility and power of the chief nursing officer.

The Job Enjoyment scale, which was developed from Brayfield and Rothe's (1951) questionnaire, is defined as follows:

- Job Enjoyment: Measure of the degree to which people like their work

The NDNQI RN Survey includes additional questions on the nursing work context and situations that occurred on the last shift. Three of these questions are addressed in this monograph, with the following response options: *strongly agree, agree, tend to agree, tend to disagree, disagree,* or *strongly disagree.*

- "Overall, I had a good day."
- "I received an orientation that adequately prepared me for my current position
- "My patient assignment was appropriate, considering both the number of patients and the care they required."

References

Aiken, L. & Patrician, P.A. (2000). Measuring organizational traits of hospitals: The Revised Nursing Work Index. *Nursing Research, 49,* 146-153.

Brayfield, A. & Rothe, H. (1951). An index of job satisfaction. *Journal of Applied Psychology, 35,* 307-311.

Stamps, P. (1997). *Nurses and work satisfaction: An index for measurement.* Chicago: Health Administration Press.

Taunton, R.L., Bott, M.J., Koehn, M.L., Miller, P., Rindner, E., Pace, K., Elliott, C., Bradley, K.J., Boyle, D., & Dunton, N. (2004). The NDNQI-Adapted Index of Work Satisfaction. *Journal of Nursing Measurement, 12,* 101-122.

Using a Shared Governance Model to Improve Nurse Job Satisfaction

Cheryl Dumont, PhD, RN
Director, Nursing Research
cdumont@valleyhealthlink.com

Kathryn Tagnesi, BSN, MS, RN, NEA-BC
Vice President of Nursing/CNO
Winchester Medical Center

Janet Nordling, MSN, RN
Director, Women and Children

Mary David, MSN, RN, CCRN, NEA-BC
Director, Heart Center

Susan Westfall, MSN, RN
Staff Nurse, Cardiovascular Intensive Care Unit

Winchester Medical Center

Editor's Pick

INSIGHTS & IDEAS FROM THIS FACILITY

Nursing leadership and staff nurses were able to track improvement in RN job satisfaction relating to the implementation of shared governance. RNs identified and resolved issues specific to their units.

Facility and Unit Summary

Facility	Winchester Medical Center (WMC)—Winchester, VA **http://www.valleyhealthlink.com/**
Facility setting	A tertiary-care, regional referral hospital of the Valley Health System in the northwestern Shenandoah Valley in rural Virginia; area served by WMC includes 17 counties and covers a 57-mile radius
Teaching status	Teaching (residency program for family practice residents)
Ownership status	Community, nonprofit hospital
Community demographics	• Winchester Medical Center, located within 100 miles of the Washington, DC, metropolitan area, serving approximately 450,000 people in the rapidly growing tri-state area of Virginia, Maryland, and West Virginia • Largest ethnic groups: Caucasian (91%), Black/African American (4.5%), and Hispanic (3.5%) • Approximately 64% of the population less than 45 years of age
Hospital-staffed beds	375
Case mix index (CMI)	1.64
Indicators used	• Cardiovascular ICU (CVSICU): RN–RN Interactions, Professional Status, Professional Development, Nursing Management, Job Enjoyment • Labor and Delivery (L&D): RN–RN Interactions, RN–MD Interactions, Professional Status, Professional Development, and Job Enjoyment
System or unit improved	• CVSICU • L&D
NDNQI® participation	Since 2005
Time frame of QI experience	2005–2007
Magnet™ status	Magnet designation awarded September 2008
Governance model	Councilor Model for Shared Governance

Awards and recognition	• Thomson (Solucient) Top 100® Hospital—2004, 2005, 2006 • HealthGrades Awards for clinical excellence—2005, 2006, 2007, 2008, 2009 • Cleverley & Associates State of the Hospital Industry Five Star Hospital List—2006 • National Research Corporation Consumer Choice Award—2006, 2007 • Organ Donation Medal of Honor from the Virginia Organ Procurement Agency—2006

UNIT PROFILES

L&D

Internal name	Labor and Delivery (L&D)
Size and type	6 L&D beds, 2 operating rooms, 3-bed post-anesthesia care unit
Staff summary	35 RNs, 5 surgical scrub technicians
Staff skill mix	Except for the operating room, 100% RN staff; 1 surgical technician scheduled per shift (during cesarean sections the technician scrubs and the RN serves as circulator)
RN-patient ratios	***Intrapartum*** 1:2 Patients in labor 1:1 Patients in second stage of labor 1:1 Patients with medical or obstetric complications 1:2 Oxytocin induction or augmentation of labor 1:1 Initiation of epidural anesthesia 1:1 Circulation for cesarean delivery ***Antepartum–postpartum*** 1:6 Antepartum and postpartum without complications 1:2 Postoperative recovery 1:3 Antepartum and postpartum with complications but stable condition 1:4 Newborns and those requiring close observation *Source:* Lockwood et al., 2007 *Note:* WMC follows the recommendations from the American Academy of Pediatrics (AAP) and the American College of Obstetricians and Gynecologists (ACOG) for staffing ratios.
Organizational structure	Vice President of Nursing, Nursing director (Women and Children's), Clinical Manager, Charge nurses

CVSICU

Internal name	Cardiovascular ICU (CVSICU)
Size and type	10 beds
Staff summary	29 RNs
Staff skill mix	100% RNs
Nurse-patient ratio (NHPPD)	1:2
Organizational structure	Vice president of nursing, nursing director (Heart Center), clinical manager, direct care nurses

Using a Shared Governance Model to Improve Nurse Job Satisfaction

Cheryl Dumont, PhD, RN
Kathryn Tagnesi, BSN, MS, RN, NEA-BC
Janet Nordling, MSN, RN
Mary David, MSN, RN, CCRN, NEA-BC
Susan Westfall, MSN, RN

Winchester Medical Center

Introductory Summary

Winchester Medical Center (WMC) is a 375-bed tertiary-care regional referral hospital in rural northwestern Virginia. This institution employs 761 bedside nurses and cares for approximately 27,000 inpatients and 213,000 outpatients annually. WMC has received the Thomson (Solucient) Top 100 Hospitals awards annually for the past 4 years, but before the journey to Magnet recognition, nursing had never been singled out for excellence.

In 2004, the vice president of nursing (VPN) introduced the concepts of shared governance and the American Nurses Credentialing Center (ANCC) journey to Magnet recognition. The process of changing the way business was conducted throughout the division of nursing began. Decision-making was moved from a top-down authoritarian approach to a shared decision-making and shared governance model. Senior leadership made it possible for change to occur through leading by example and placing the right leaders in the right places.

WMC employed the Councilor Model for Shared Governance (Foster, 1992). This model included five housewide councils: (1) Coordinating Council, (2) Leadership Council, (3) Performance Improvement Council, (4) Practice Council, and (5) Education Council (see Figure 1). Each council had representation from direct care nurses across the division of nursing, and each nursing unit created its own unit-based council (UBC). Decisions regarding nursing housewide were made by the housewide councils, while 90% of decisions regarding direct care were made at the UBC level.

During this time nursing leadership was reorganized to create a flat hierarchy. There were 21 nurse directors and no other administrative level between the approximately 750 bedside nurses and 200 non-bedside nurses and the VPN in most units. The exceptions were some units in the Heart Center, the Women and Children's Department, the Surgical Services Department, and the Emergency Department. In those cases there were large numbers of staff and clinical specialties to be coordinated; therefore, a clinical manager and/or charge nurses were employed (see Figure 2).

FIGURE 1.
The WMC Councilor Model of Shared Governance

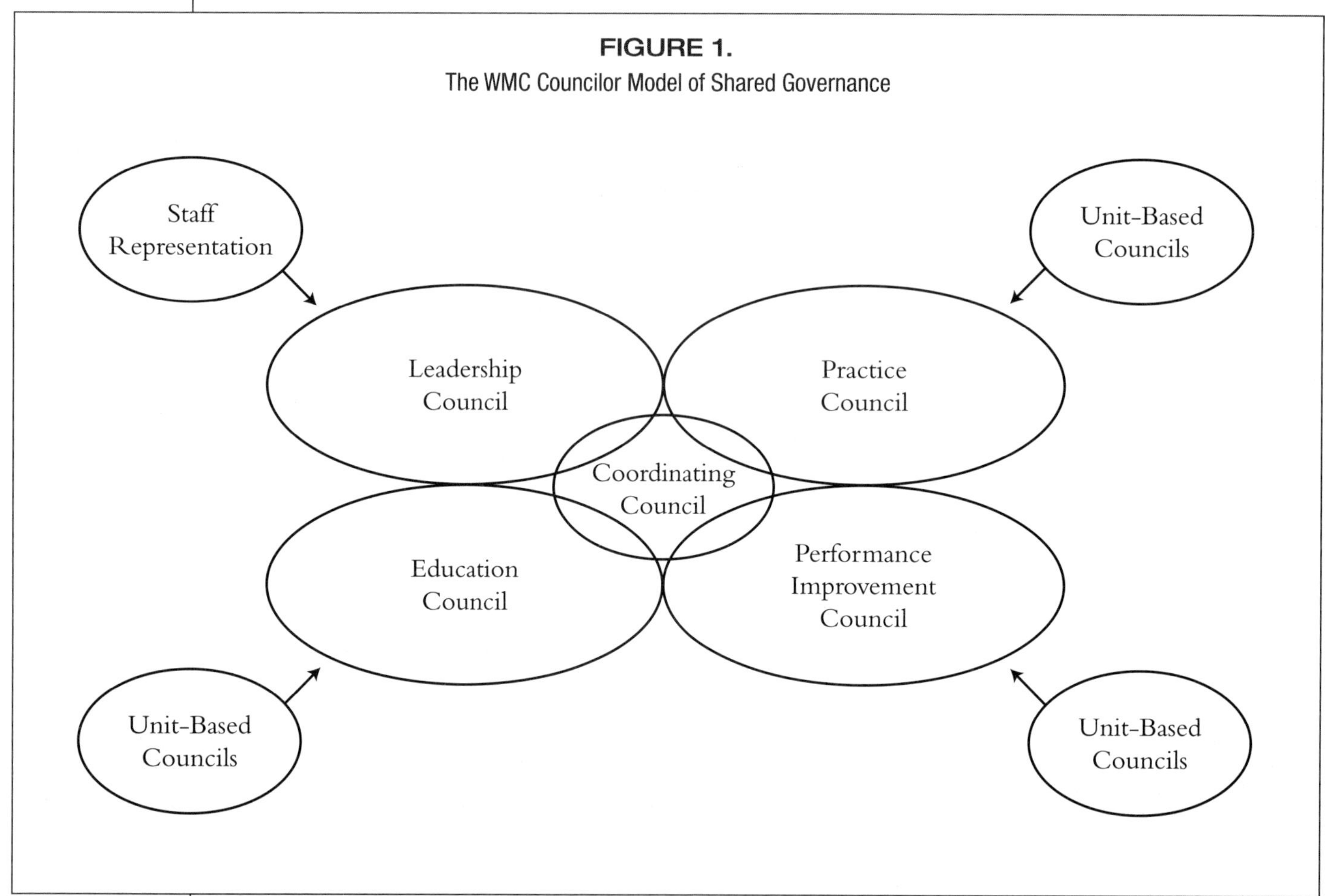

By 2005, WMC was a National Database for Nursing Quality Indicators® (NDNQI) participant hospital, and in August of that year WMC nurses participated in their first NDNQI RN Satisfaction Survey. The NDNQI RN Survey with Job Satisfaction Scales became an important part of the Magnet journey, as it provided WMC with pertinent information on nurses' satisfaction with their work environment. The 2005 results revealed that nurses at WMC were moderately satisfied with their jobs. The WMC overall job enjoyment score in 2005 was 45.5. A score of 40 to 60 was considered to be moderate satisfaction, and a score greater than 60 was considered high satisfaction. While a score of 45.5 was not a bad score, it did not reflect the excellent environment envisioned by the nurses. In response, the nursing leaders and staff carefully reviewed results of the RN survey, and the questions from each subscale, at their UBC meetings. Action plans were then created and initiatives established based on their insights. By 2006, the average WMC nursing unit job enjoyment score had improved to 50. In 2007, the average score was 49, with some units reaching scores in the 60s. While there still is work to be done, it has been gratifying to have seen progress in many of the nursing units.

Combining of Unit-Based Decision-Making and NDNQI Results

The driving forces behind the improvements in nursing job enjoyment were changes in leadership style and the institution of a shared governance and shared decision-making model. Within the structure of this model, the results of the RN survey were shared with nursing leadership who, in turn, reviewed the results

FIGURE 2.
WMC Nursing Organizational Chart

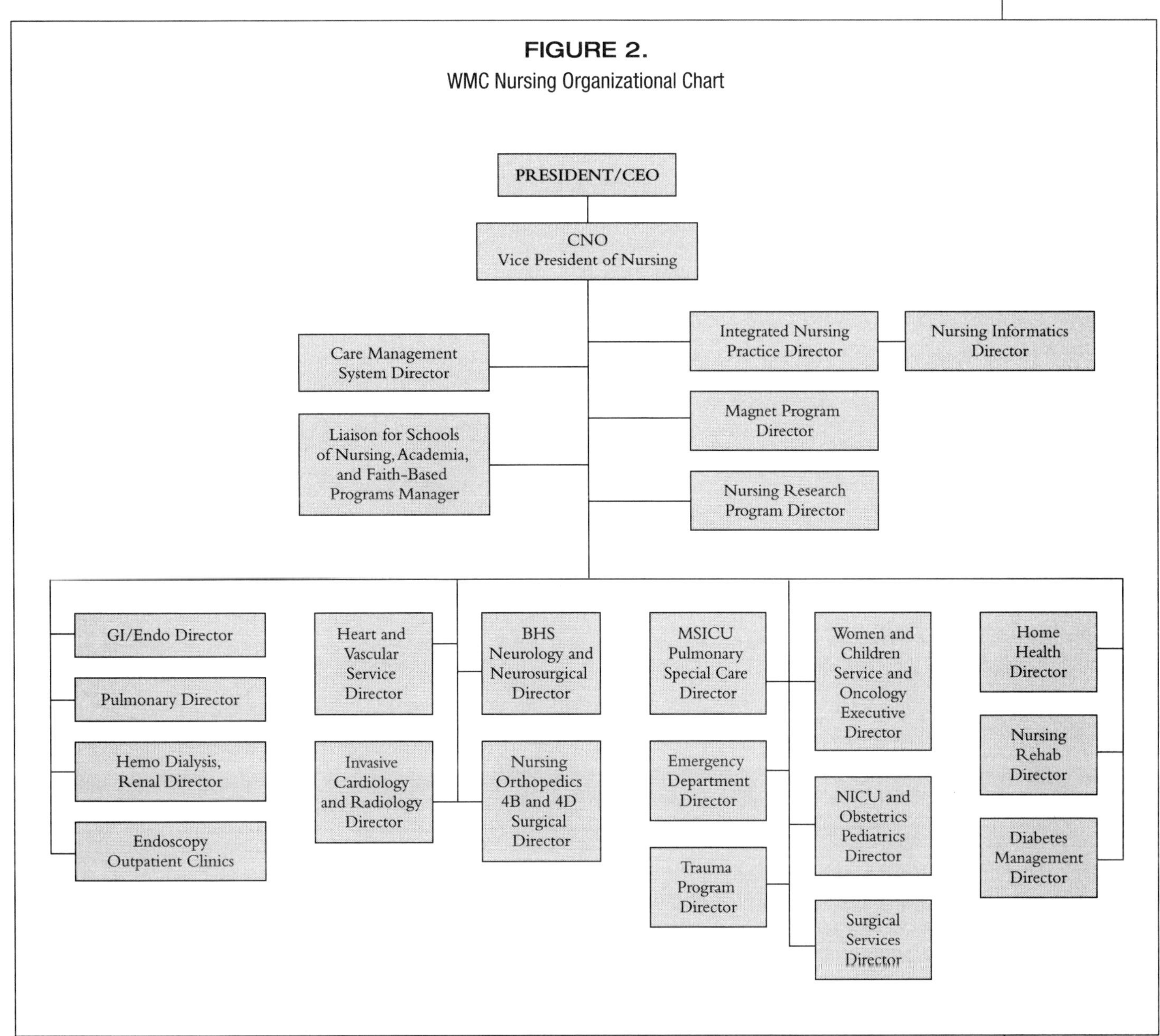

with their unit-based council members and all other staff. Each unit was able to identify the areas in most need of improvement and work to develop solutions and interventions. The following paragraphs provide exemplars from two units demonstrating how the NDNQI data were used at the unit level to guide interventions for improvement in the work environment and job enjoyment. L&D and the CVSICU have shown sustained improvement in nurse job enjoyment.

Individual Unit Examples

Labor and Delivery Unit's RN–MD Interactions

The first NDNQI RN Satisfaction Survey was performed in August 2005. The initial results were received in October and were first shared with the staff in the December staff meetings. In 2005, the L&D unit had a poor job enjoyment score (38.68) and an even worse RN–MD interaction score (26.43).

The staff were well aware that interdisciplinary interactions had been identified as important, not only to individual job satisfaction but also to patient outcomes (Fewster-Thuente & Velsor-Friedrich, 2008; TJC, 2008). They also were aware and concerned that their relationships with the WMC physicians were not conducive to good communication and teamwork. The NDNQI data provided concrete evidence that the majority of the nurses felt the same way and wanted to do something about it.

During the first quarter of 2006, the L&D nurses researched the issue and formulated a plan. One underlying problem identified in the literature was the difference between the perceptions of physicians and nurses of the significance of their interactions. For example, in response to the question "How do you rate physician value and respect for nurse input and collaboration?" Rosenstein identified that on a scale of 1 to 10, with 10 being strongest agreement, the mean nurse rating was 5.83 (N = 716, SD = 2.2) and the mean physician rating was 7.26 (N = 173, SD = 1.8) ($p < 0.001$). Thus, physicians perceived their behaviors to be more respectful of the nurses than the nurses perceived those same behaviors. The study also demonstrated that physicians rated the seriousness of disruptive physician behavior lower than nurses rated it, that is, 5.96 versus 7.13, with $p < 0.001$ (Rosenstein, 2002).

There are many reasons why physicians and nurses differed on perceptions of their interactions. These reasons include gender differences, cultural differences, and hierarchy and power in relationships (Casanova, Davy & Dorpat, 2007; Coombs & Ersser, 2004). However, with this understanding, the L&D nurses decided the first step would be to find out what the perceptions were between the two disciplines on L&D and to raise awareness with the results. They would start with a survey of the physicians and nurses to determine what they perceived to be the major issues.

By the second quarter 2006, the WMC nursing administrators met with the medical director and the medical department chair to discuss the problem and present their plan. The physicians were distressed that the nurses had rated their RN–MD interactions so poorly and were in agreement with the plan for a survey.

The survey employed a qualitative method, asking two open-ended questions. The L&D staff had used this method previously when looking at improving the relationship between the night shift staff on the L&D unit and the Mother/Baby unit. The method led to information that was successfully employed in improving the relationship between the two groups. The two open-ended questions asked were (1) What promotes collegial relationships? and (2) What hinders collegial relationships?

The survey met the criteria for WMC Institutional Review Board exempt status because it was anonymous and voluntary. The surveys were distributed to 15 physicians and 33 nurses. The response rate was 60% (9) for the physicians and 45% (15) for the nurses. The responses were analyzed for themes and a list was developed of the top 10 most commonly mentioned behaviors for each question (see Table 1). The major themes were communication and respect.

After analysis the nurses met with the obstetric (OB) physicians to present the results. Each member of the team agreed to make efforts to promote positive behaviors and decrease the hindering behaviors. They also explored other areas that could be improved, with much of the discussion focused on how difficult it is for the nursing staff when there is a lack of standardization in physician practice. The nurses identified evidence that standardization improves outcomes in highly complex organizations such as healthcare (Welch, 2007). The physicians agreed that there were many practices that could easily become standardized, and consensus was achieved to proceed in that direction.

The unit-based practice council worked with the medical director and the department chair to get the ball rolling. Over the next 3 years the unit successfully standardized many practices, such as the surgi-

TABLE 1.
RN–MD Interactions Survey for the Labor and Delivery Unit

Top 10 Things That Promote and Hinder Collegial Relationships between RNs and MDs

	Promotes		Hinders	
	Physician response	*Nurse response*	*Physician response*	*Nurse response*
1	Respect	Respect	Excessive workloads, space constraints, limited staffing	Condescending remarks, "holier than thou" attitudes
2	Communication	Communication	No sense of humor	Verbal abuse of RN by MD in front of patients
3	Humor	Standard practice among MDs	Lack of respect for other person's knowledge	MDs bringing personal problems to work
4	Courtesy "Thank you"	Teamwork	Laziness, poor patient care, inattentiveness	Poor verbal communication (that is, mumbling, incomplete thoughts)
5	Teamwork	MD education for RNs	Sarcastic attitudes	Lack of trust
6	Good patient care, good case/status presentations	MD appreciation of nurses' role	Gossip, social gatherings in nurses' station	Nurses being caught in MD-to-MD issue or MD-to-patient issue
7	Professional behavior of RNs	Putting patients first	Favoritism to certain doctors	MDs' unkind gossip about other nurses
8	RNs keeping private lives private	Professionalism	MDs' poor anger management	"Testing" of new nurses
9	Consideration, empathy, compassion for each other	Trust	Refusal to follow orders	MD annoyance when called with patient issues or a new patient
10	Rounding	MD responding to nurses' concerns, being available	Lack of consideration	Inconsistent practices among MDs

cal prep used for C-section patients, L&D admission orders, vaginal and C-section postpartum physician orders, delivery-recovery orders, preoperative anti biotic administration, high- and low-dose regimens for Pitocin administration, and the Cervidil order set. After successfully standardizing order sets with the OB physicians, the practice council then worked with the anesthesiologist group and successfully standardized the epidural infusion order set as well.

By August 2007, the L&D RN–MD interaction scores had increased dramatically, from 26.43 to 47.68. The job enjoyment score increased from 38.68 in 2005 to 53.63 (Figure 3). The L&D unit also made improvements on every subscale of the RN survey and scored in the top quartile on two subscales (RN–RN interactions and professional development; Figure 4).

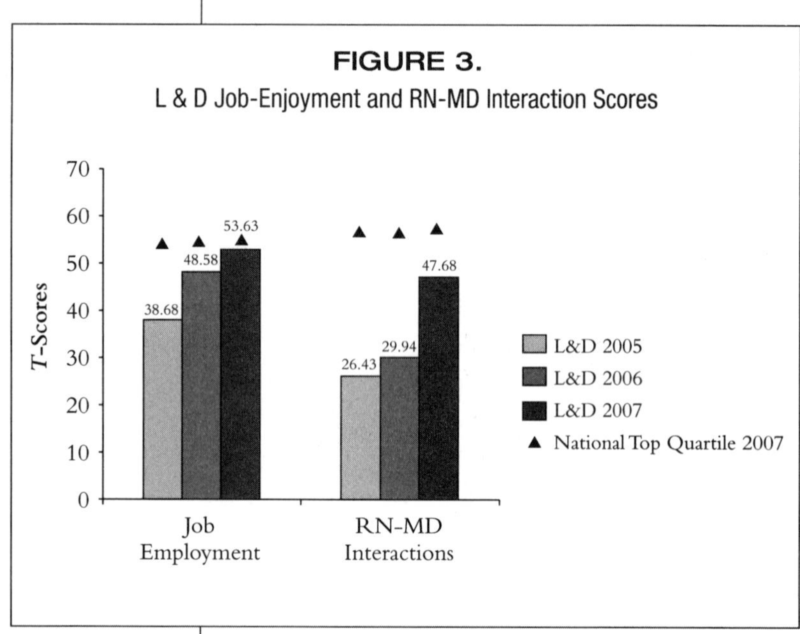

FIGURE 3.
L & D Job-Enjoyment and RN-MD Interaction Scores

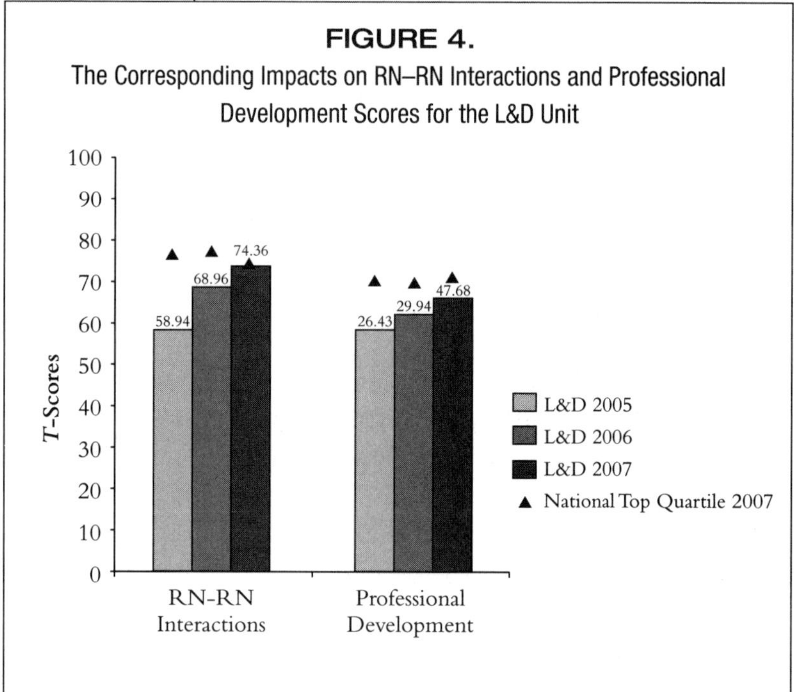

FIGURE 4.
The Corresponding Impacts on RN–RN Interactions and Professional Development Scores for the L&D Unit

The L&D staff and OB physicians were excited to see the increased scores for RN–MD interactions, but were not surprised. Members of both disciplines verbalized experiencing a difference in the relationships. There was a significant decrease in the number of complaints made to the director by the staff and physicians about each other. In addition, after standardizing the antibiotic prep and the surgical prep, the C-section infection rate fell from 2.7% in 2006 to zero in 2008. The nurse vacancy rate declined from 2% in 2006 to 0% in 2008.

Cardiovascular Intensive Care Unit

The CVSICU has been an exemplary unit with regard to nurse satisfaction. The unit showed improvement in all 11 subscales over the past 3 years. Seven of their 11 subscales for satisfaction were at or above the NDNQI comparison top quartile in 2007 (see Figure 5). The highest scoring subscales in 2007 were satisfaction with RN–RN interactions (66.39), professional status (68.92), professional development (68.92), and satisfaction with nursing management (61.07). Two other subscales with improvements were decision-making (54.95) and autonomy (55.71). The effect of improvement in all scores is reflected in the dramatic increase in the job enjoyment score, from 44.58 in 2005 to 57.67 in 2007. This improvement in satisfaction was a result of initiatives driven by the staff members as well as the supervision and leadership of a new nursing unit director. The initiatives, presented in the following paragraphs, include the institution of a new leadership style, development of shared decision-making through unit-based councils, an emphasis on professional development, and a mentoring program developed by the staff themselves.

Mentorship program and RN–RN interactions

The CVSICU turned around its reputation from a unit that "eats their young," demonstrated by a lack of nurse teamwork, collegiality, and support of new staff in 2005, to a unit known for excellent RN–RN interactions in 2007 (56.06 versus 66.39). This improvement in RN–RN interactions was in large part due to the institution of the staff-led mentor program and redesign of the unit orientation process. The staff members noted that scores were low in this area and felt that they needed to take a look at themselves and how new people were accepted into the unit and supported throughout their stay.

FIGURE 5.

Work in Shared Governance and Mentoring That Improved Scores across the Board for CVSICU

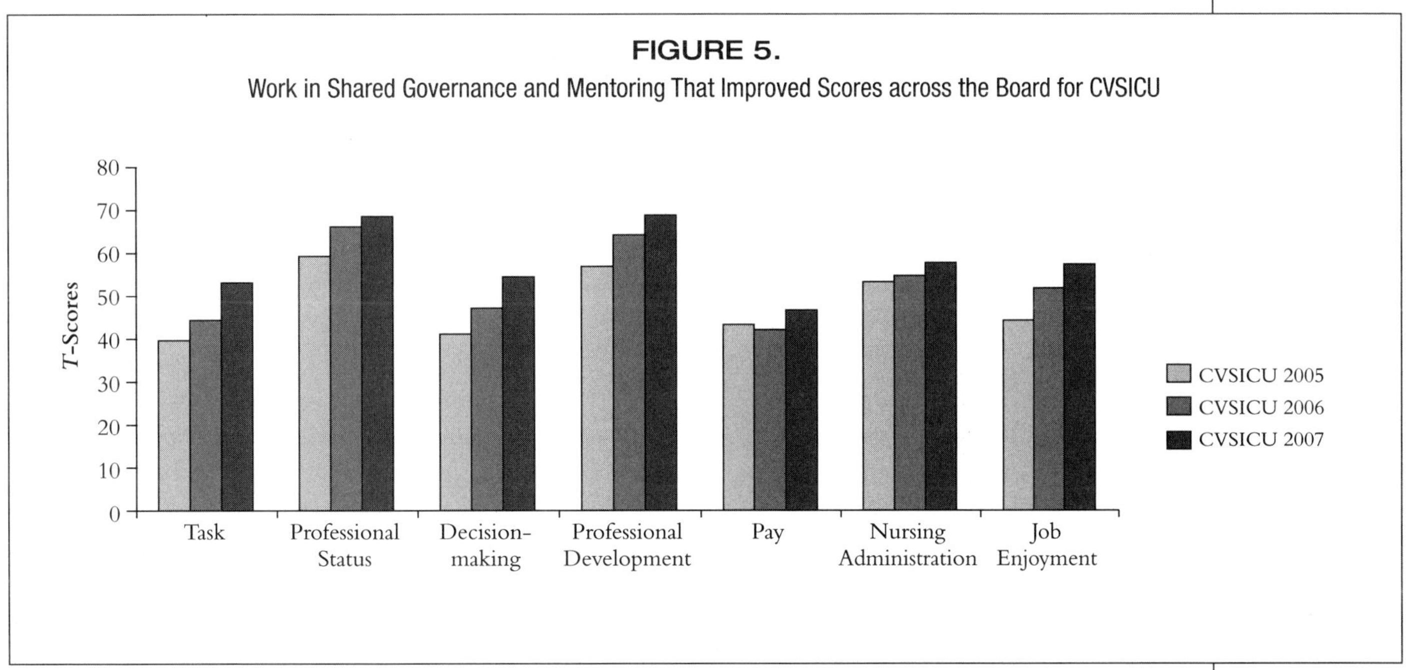

Ideas for a mentor program were brought back by a staff nurse as an evidence-based best practice from the TRENDS in Critical Care Conference, sponsored by the Southeastern Pennsylvania Chapter of the American Association of Critical Care Nurses in April 2006. One of the sessions staff attended was titled "The Art of Mentoring," presented by Amy Funderburk, MSN, RN, CNA. A literature review was performed, and criteria for selection of both mentors and mentees were developed by the staff using information from experts in the field (Dorsey & Baker, 2004; Funderburk, 2008; Sherwen, 2007; Zachary, 2007). The program was based on developing relationships and provided support for new staff in many ways. It has been very successful in improving RN–RN interactions and decreasing nurse turnover. Currently all RN positions are filled, and the last new hire was chosen from seven applicants for the position.

Nursing management

In 2006, the CVSICU gained a new clinical director. The director supported the staff in their initiatives for shared governance and in allocation of funds from the budget for work in research, performance improvement, and educational opportunities.

Choosing new staff members was a critical decision that affected the functioning and morale of the whole team. Staff nurses provided valuable insight into the needs of the unit as well as the characteristics in potential new staff that would meet those needs. The nursing director facilitated staff discussion and input into the selection criteria for new hires and ensured staff nurse representation on the interview teams of potential new hires. This process has engendered a feeling of cohesiveness among the staff and more staff involvement in the functioning of the unit. The result has been improved satisfaction with nursing management, from a score of 43.95 in 2005 to 61.07 in 2007.

Professional development and professional status

There has been an increased use of evidence-based practice, a higher value placed on education and scholarly activities, and recognition for staff demonstration of excellence in the CVSICU. Shared decision-making through the shared governance councilor model was embraced in this unit. Nurses tackled a number of issues within the structure of their unit-based practice and education councils. One project involved collaboration with the cardiovascular (CV) surgeons to create a CV protocol book. The book is evidence based and has standardized practice in the unit to be best practice. The development and implementation of the book has given the nurses a great sense of self-worth and of proving value to the healthcare system.

The CVSICU professional development score improved from 57.44 in 2005 to 69.10 in 2007, due in large part to the push by the unit director for nurses to become proactive in their own development and to attend conferences and seminars outside the organization. The education council was given authority by the unit director to determine what the educational needs were and how to best allocate budgeted funds. From 2006 through 2007, 21 of 29 staff nurses were funded to attend educational conferences, both locally and nationally.

All staff sponsored to go to conferences were responsible for bringing information back to the unit. For example, a staff nurse brought back information on a computerized insulin dose calculator for tight glycemic control. The unit had been struggling with this issue, and the information helped lead to a randomized controlled trial designed by a team of staff nurses and the director of nursing research. Other examples of projects developed through shared governance council work and professional development of the nurses were a protocol for hypothermia in postarrest patients and the development of a rapid response team.

The staff also supported each other to achieve national certification in critical care nursing, with a goal of 100% certification for those eligible. In the past year, the CVSICU increased the percentage of eligible critical care registered nurses (CCRNs) from 32% to 57%. In addition to encouraging and helping each other study, staff nurses created a "Wall of Honor" just inside the entryway to the unit. This wall showcases for families, visitors, and other disciplines all the nurses who have achieved national certification. Many members of the CVSICU also were actively involved in and support the newly revitalized local chapter of AACN. A staff nurse from CVSICU is the current chapter president.

Conclusions and Implications

Visionary leadership, a shared decision-making, shared governance model, and the ability to track the effects of new initiatives through the NDNQI and to identify trends have been the key ingredients in the improvements in nurse job enjoyment. The members of the board of directors of WMC were successful in choosing a creative and visionary nursing leader, who put in place a team of creative, visionary, and motivated nursing directors at the unit level. The chief nurse supported and guided the directors to lead their staffs through the difficult organizational changes to achieve higher levels of professionalism with a shared governance model and use of evidence-based practice. The chief nurse also had the foresight to enroll WMC nursing in the NDNQI to provide a tracking and benchmarking mechanism. Staff nurses rose to the occasion and accepted the accountability that comes with increased decision-making power. The WMC transformation started with a few exceptional nurses leading the way for many who were hopeful, some who were indifferent, and a few who were strong naysayers. The successes outweighed the failures and persistence paid off. Today WMC is a very exciting and rewarding place for a nurse to work.

Two implications for future practice are evident. First, the successes experienced by the nurses in the L&D unit and CVSICU can serve as a model for other nursing units. Demonstration of the gains in the NDNQI RN Satisfaction Survey sources and the real-life testimony of peers have been a tipping point for culture change at WMC. Nurses from these two units and other units successful in shared governance initiatives are the best mentors and leaders for others struggling to implement an environment of excellence in health care.

Second, leadership now has a better understanding of the power of shared governance and the use of comparative databases. Research has demonstrated that simply monitoring comparative data for a metric can affect its performance (Advisory Board Company,

2006). Therefore, the next logical step is to combine the strategy of shared governance, professional nurse empowerment, and use of comparative databases to affect outcomes for all the key nurse-sensitive metrics in health care.

References

Advisory Board Company. (2006). *The data-driven nursing enterprise. Leveraging data to advance hospital nursing.* Nursing Executive Center, The Advisory Board Company, Washington, DC.

Casanova, J., Davy, K., & Dorpat, D. (2007). Nurse-physician work relations and role Expectations. *JONA, 37*(2), 68–70.

Coombs, M., & Ersser, S. J. (2004). Medical hegemony in decision-making: A barrier to interdisciplinary working in intensive care? *Journal of Advanced Nursing, 46*(3), 245–252.

Dorsey, L. E., & Baker, C. M. (2004). Mentoring undergraduate nursing students. Assessing the state of the science. *Nurse Educator, 29*(6), 260–265.

Fewster-Thuente, L., & Velsor-Friedrich, B. (2008). Interdisciplinary collaboration for healthcare professionals. *Nursing Administration Quarterly, 32*(1), 40–48.

Foster, B. E. (1992). Models of shared governance: Design and implementation. In T. Porter-O'Grady (Ed.), *Implementing shared governance. Creating a professional organization* (pp. 79–110). Baltimore: Mosby.

Funderburk, A. E. (2008). Mentoring. The retention factor in the acute care setting. *Journal for Nurses in Staff Development, 24*(3), E1–E5.

The Joint Commission (TJC). (2008). Sentinel event alert. Behaviors that undermine a culture of safety. Retrieved July 29, 2008, from http://www.jointcommission.org/SentinelEvents/SentinelEventAlert/sea_40.htm

Lockwood, C., et.al. (Eds.). (2007). *Guidelines for perinatal care, 6th Edition.* Elk Grove, IL: American Academy of Pediatrics; Washington, DC: American College of Obstetricians and Gynecologists.

Rosenstein, A. H. (2002). Nurse-physician relationship: Impact on nurse satisfaction and retention. *American Journal of Nursing,* 102(6), 26–34.

Sherwen, L. N. (2007). Finding a mentor: What every nursing student should know. *Nursing Resources.* Retrieved April 7, 2007, from http://www/nso.com/resources/studartcls_mentor.php

Welch, S. J. (2007). Managing critical issues: Leading physicians through change. *Emergency Medicine News, 29*(8), 22–23.

Zachary, L. J. (2007). Creating a mentoring culture. Retrieved April 7, 2007, from http://humanresources.about.com/od/coachingmentoring/a/mentor_culture.htm

Sustained Improvement in RN Satisfaction Measures: "Overall Had a Good Day" as an Indicator of a Positive Nurse Environment

Madeline Albanese, RN, MSN
Manager, Nursing Performance Improvement
Madeline.albanese@uphs.upenn.edu

Sandra Dietrich, RN, MSN, MHA
Director, Emergency Services

Leigh Ann Schmidt, RN, BSN
Nurse Manager, Emergency Nursing

Kathlyn Schumacher, RN, MSN, CRNP
Nurse Practitioner, Clinical and Translational Research Center

A. Lorraine Norfleet, RN, BSN, MHA
Nurse Manager, Clinical and Translational Research Center

Noreen McHugh, RN, MSN
Clinical Director, Perioperative Nursing

Marianne Saunders, RN, BSN
Nurse Manager, OR South

Marie Zubko, RN, BSN
Nurse Manager, OR Blue

Victoria L. Rich, PhD, RN, FAAN
Chief Nursing Executive
University of Pennsylvania Medical Center

Sandra Jost, MSN, RN
Associate Chief Nursing Officer

Hospital of the University of Pennsylvania

Editor's Pick

INSIGHTS & IDEAS FROM THIS FACILITY

"Backcasting" helped units create a vision of a better nursing work environment. The plan to achieve this vision led to improved RN satisfaction and reduced turnover.

Facility and Unit Summary

Facility	Hospital of the University of Pennsylvania—Philadelphia, Pennsylvania **www.pennhealth.com**
Facility setting	Urban
Teaching status	Academic medical center
Ownership status	Nonprofit
Community demographics	• Urban setting in West Philadelphia within Philadelphia metropolitan region • 75% of patients reside within the city, and surrounding and outlying counties • Approximately 14% of service area population over age 65
Hospital-staffed beds	623
Case mix index (CMI)	2.25
System or unit improved	• OR Blue • OR South • Emergency Department (ED) • Clinical and Translational Research Center (CTRC)
Indicator(s) improved	RN satisfaction—Overall Had a Good Day
NDNQI® participation	Since 2004
Magnet™ status	First designation June 2007
Governance model	Nursing Shared Governance
Awards and recognition	• U.S. News and World Report Best Hospitals Honor Roll (ranked 10th in 2008) • American Association of Critical Care Nurses Beacon Award • Surgical Critical Care Units: Rhoads 5 Surgical Critical Care, SICU-Cardiothoracic, SICU-Neurotrauma • Progressive Care Unit: Silverstein 10 (Cardiothoracic Surgery) • Hospitals and Health Networks Most Wired Hospitals (2008) • American Alliance of Healthcare Providers Hospital of Choice Awards

UNIT PROFILES

OR BLUE

Internal name	OR Blue
Size and type	Average: 13 operating rooms/day
Staff summary	34 registered nurses; 21 surgical technicians
Staff skill mix	60% RNs
Nurse-patient ratio (NHPPD)	Not applicable
Organizational structure	Nurse manager, Clinical nurses, Surgical technicians

OR SOUTH

Internal name	OR South
Size and type	8 operating rooms; cardiac, thoracic, vascular, and transplant services
Staff summary	30 registered nurses; 13 surgical technicians
Staff skill mix	60% RN
Nurse-patient ratio (NHPPD)	Not applicable)
Organizational structure	Nurse manager, clinical nurses, surgical technicians

ED

Internal name	Emergency Department
Size and type	25 general care beds, 3 trauma beds, 6 fast-track beds, and 8 Clinical Decision Unit beds; emergency medicine
Staff summary	90 RNs; 23 ED technicians; 16 emergency medical technicians (EMTs)
Staff skill mix	70% RNs
Nurse-patient ratio (NHPPD)	1:5
Organizational structure	Nurse manager, Assistant nurse manager, Clinical nurses, Emergency technicians

CTRC

Internal name	Clinical and Translational Research Center (CTRC)
Size and type	8 inpatient beds, 11 outpatient spaces; core facility for patient-related clinical research
Staff summary	11 RNs, 1 medical technician
Staff skill mix	90% RNs
Nurse–patient ratio (NHPPD)	Not applicable
Organizational structure	Nurse Manager, Clinical Nurses, Research technicians

Sustained Improvement in RN Satisfaction Measures: "Overall Had a Good Day" as an Indicator of a Positive Nurse Environment

Madeline Albanese, RN, MSN
Sandra Dietrich, RN, MSN, MHA
Leigh Ann Schmidt, RN, BSN
Kathlyn Schumacher, RN, MSN, CRNP
A. Lorraine Norfleet, RN, BSN, MHA
Noreen McHugh, RN, MSN
Marianne Saunders, RN, BSN
Marie Zubko, RN, BSN
Victoria L. Rich, PhD, RN, FAAN
Sandra Jost, MSN, RN

Hospital of the University of Pennsylvania

Introductory Summary

The Hospital of the University of Pennsylvania (HUP) is a 704-bed (623 staffed beds) academic medical center located in West Philadelphia. The hospital primarily serves adults and includes a Level 1 Trauma Center (approximately 2,500 trauma cases/year), a Level 3 Intensive Care Nursery; 32 operating rooms (approximately 24,000 cases/year); a robust transplantation program; high-volume oncology, cardiology, and hospitalist services; and a busy emergency department (approximately 59,000 visits/FY 2007). The nursing division at HUP is composed of approximately 1,700 RNs, approximately 88% of whom hold a BSN or higher nursing degree.

HUP clinical nurses have participated in the National Database of Nursing Indicators® (NDNQI) RN satisfaction survey for 4 consecutive years. Average unit response rate each year from 2004 to 2007 ranged from 76% to 84% (representing 1,102 to 1,404 respondents). Participation is highly valued and supported by all levels of hospital and nursing leadership. Results are shared at all levels, from clinical nurses at the bedside to the board of trustees. Findings are reviewed intensively and acted upon in the ensuing year through hospital, divisional, and unit-level forums. The chief nurse executive prepares an annual summary of initiatives for the past year—titled "You responded and here's what we did"—based on feedback from the previous year's survey results. Data related to RN–MD relation-

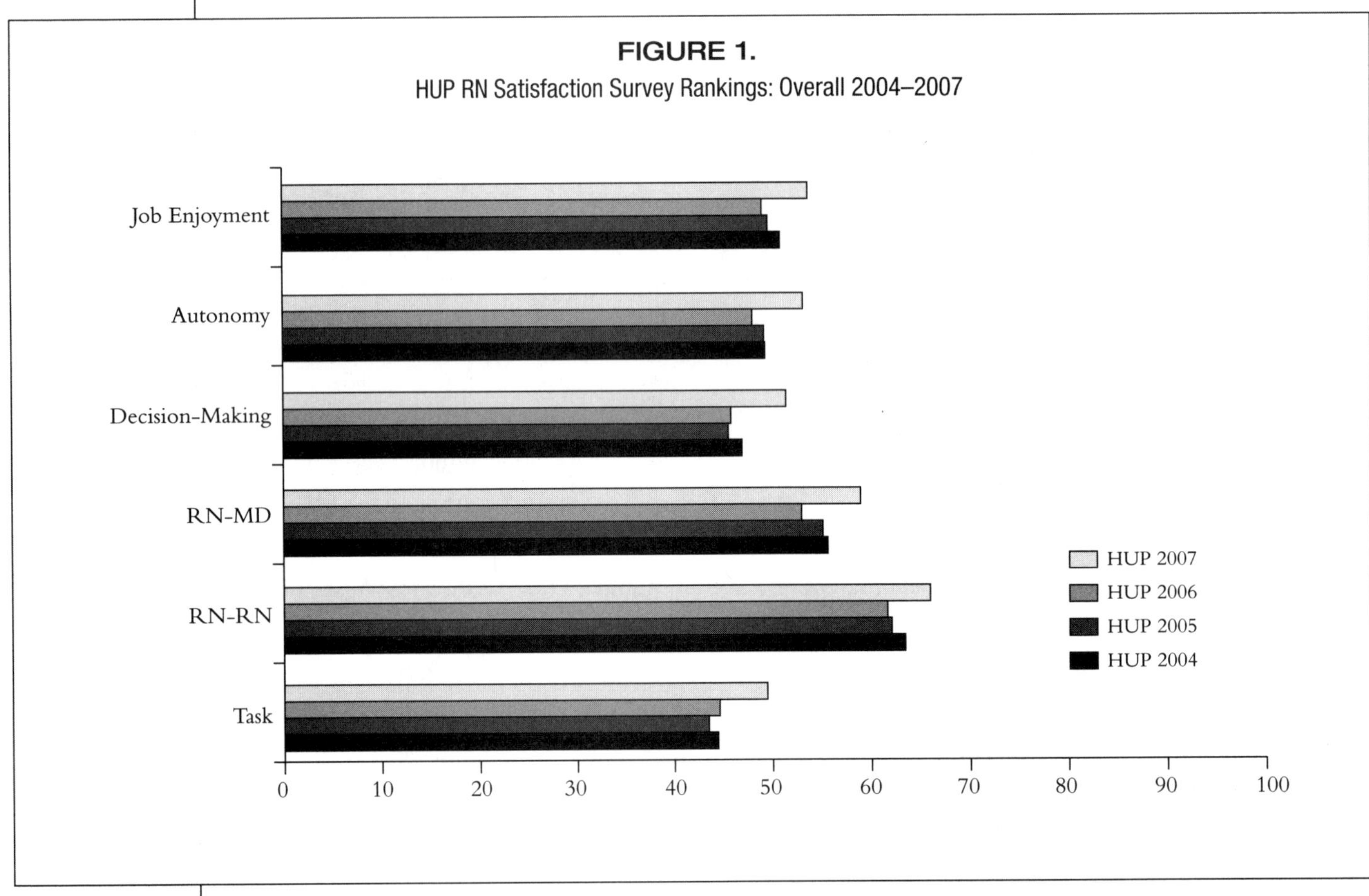

ships are shared with and considered in department chairs' evaluations.

The impact of HUP's journey to Magnet™ and subsequent designation in June 2007 has been reflected in higher ratings of satisfaction by HUP's clinical nurses. From 2004 to 2007, HUP clinical nurses reported varying degrees of satisfaction during the transformation of the culture and establishment of the shared governance model. In 2007, the hospitalwide results demonstrated that HUP nurses were moderately to highly satisfied in all measures of the Adapted Index of Work Satisfaction (see Figure 1). Satisfaction scores in all of these measures also had improved over 2006 scores and were significantly above the mean of the 2007 NDNQI comparison group in all measures except RN–RN relationships and job enjoyment. HUP scores related to satisfaction with professional development were in the top quartile of the 2007 NDNQI comparison group data.

The increase in satisfaction measures reported by HUP clinical nurses also was reflected in the responses to the work contextual item, "rating of the last shift"—specifically, "Overall had a good day." In 2007, HUP nurses reported a satisfaction rating of 4.42 on a scale of 1 to 6 (with 1 being "strongly disagree" and 6 being "strongly agree"), up from a rating of 4.22 in 2006 (see Figure 2). This article highlights how advances in the nursing work environment contributed to a sustained increase of the nurses' ratings of "Overall had a good day" in the Emergency Department, OR Blue, OR South, and the Clinical and Translational Research Center.

Experiences and Consequences

HUP clinical nurses have participated in the NDNQI RN satisfaction survey each September or October for 4 consecutive years, beginning in 2004.

Survey results are shared with unit leadership, including the unit council chair, nurse manager, assistant nurse manager, and clinical nurse specialist. Graphical data displays and Excel tables are prepared for each unit and are reviewed and discussed at unit council and staff meetings. If the data show deterioration in satisfaction for any survey measure, the unit council chair and nurse manager collaboratively develop an action plan. A significant decrease is indicated when a score is below the national confidence interval limit. Comparison data are used for the national norm that coincides with the practice specialty. Action plans must include a detailed description of all action steps and measurable outcomes for each action. These action plans are forwarded to the clinical directors for review, and the outcomes defined in these plans are incorporated into the performance expectation for clinical directors and nurse managers.

FIGURE 2.
HUP RN Satisfaction: Overall Had a Good Day, Mean Values 2004–2007

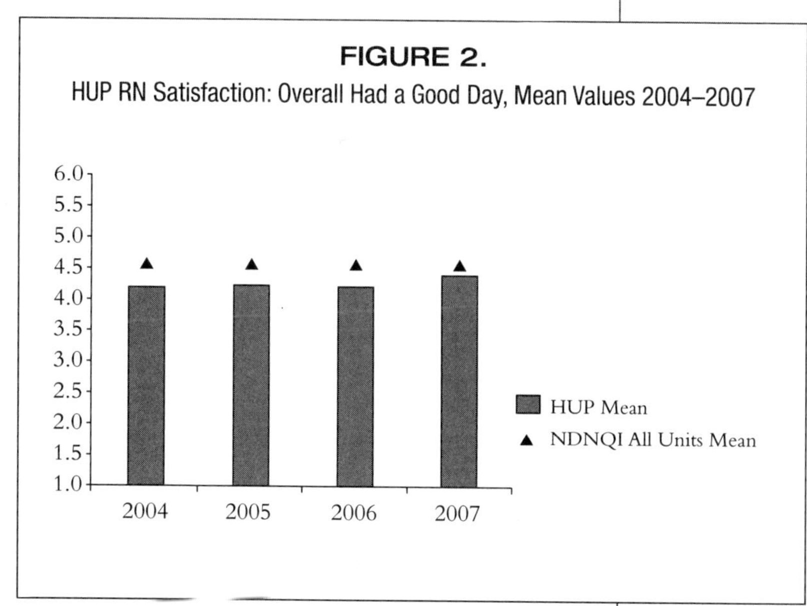

Over the years of participation in the RN satisfaction survey and the journey to Magnet designation, the department has experienced several challenges in improving the nurse work environment, retaining nurses, and enhancing their job satisfaction. The challenge to transform the culture was met through several related initiatives, including the introduction of the HUP Nursing Excellence in Professional Practice™ model and the Nursing Shared Governance model.

The HUP Nursing Excellence in Professional Practice model is structured as a three-dimensional pyramid circumscribed by three principles that need to be ever-present if high-quality patient care is to be achieved and maintained (see Figure 3). These principles are a respectful workplace, collaboration, and skilled communication. The professional practice model delineates the remaining 11 components as building upon one another in a complex, stepwise fashion with the suggestion that the depth, breadth, and height of each principle are constantly in flux but always interconnected. The integration of this model with the strategic direction of the organization and national nursing standards is reflected by the University of Pennsylvania Health System Core Values on the right side of the model, an adaptation of the American Association of Critical Care Nurse Standards for Healthy Work Environments (2005), and the Nursing Organization Alliance Principles and Elements of a Healthful Practice/Work Environment (2004).

The Integrated Primary Nursing (IPN) Delivery Care Model is a balanced blend of Marie Manthey's Primary and Relationship-Based Care Models (1984 and 2004, respectively). The foundation of HUP's nursing practice is found in relationships developed between the patient/family and nurse, through which all healthcare needs are met and preferences for care and diversity are respected. The IPN model embraces the recent trends in health care of higher acuity, episodic patient encounters, and technological advancements. The integrated primary nurse adheres to five tenets for nursing practice: patient- and family-focused, evidence-based, accountable, coordinated, and continuous. The unit councils are accountable to design care based on the tenets of the practice model, to ensure that individual patient outcomes are maximized. The World Class Patient Care and Integrated Primary Nursing models cannot evolve beyond the baseline of structure, process, outcome, and life-long learning without an organizational culture that supports authentic leadership, shared governance, partnership, evidence-based practice, translational research, and innovation In addition, without the foundational principles of respectful

FIGURE 3.
HUP Nursing Excellence in Professional Practice

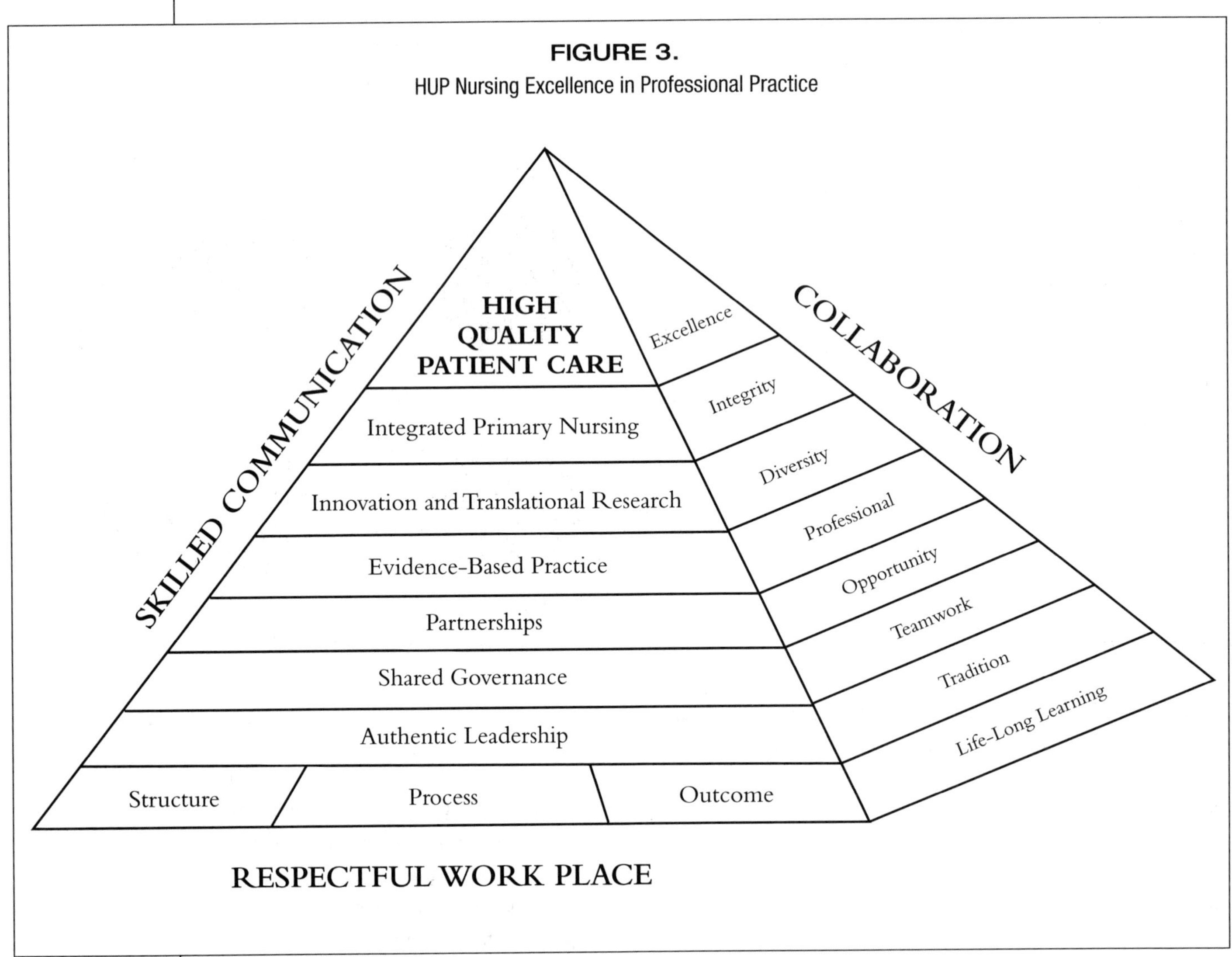

workplace, skilled communication, and collaboration, nursing care cannot be effectively practiced.

The HUP Nursing Shared Governance model (see Figure 4) provides the framework for a participative practice environment that values clinical nurse input and feedback. The structure of unit councils, core councils, and the Nursing Shared Governance Leadership Council provide avenues for clinical nurses to help shape their practice and influence decisions in the department.

Unit councils—each chaired by a clinical nurse and composed of clinical nurses, a support-staff representative, a nurse manager, and a clinical nurse specialist—serve as forums for communication and decision-making about unit-specific issues and concerns. Standing agenda items—practice, quality, stewardship, and professional development—ensure communication and discussion of Core Council issues. Unit council members are responsible for sharing discussions and outcomes with their unit colleagues.

To ensure that clinical nurses are able to provide leadership and express their opinions, ideas, and recommendations, they are members of the Core Councils for practice, quality, stewardship, and professional development. Councils function autonomously, and each council is able to work with other councils to achieve mutual goals. Core Councils are cochaired by a member of the nursing leadership team and a clinical nurse. Membership includes clinical nurses from a cross-section of units, to ensure representation for clinical specialization and various practice settings.

The Nursing Shared Governance Leadership Council, chaired by the chief nurse executive or associate chief nursing officer (ACNO) and a clinical nurse, is composed of the unit council chairs (clinical nurses), Core Council cochairs, and the nurse executive team (clinical directors). The Nursing Shared Governance Leadership Council serves as the collective voice for nursing in making department-level decisions, and provides an important communication link between the core councils and unit councils, as well as with nursing leadership and hospital administrators. These relationships allow bidirectional communication.

FIGURE 4.
HUP Nursing Shared Governance Model

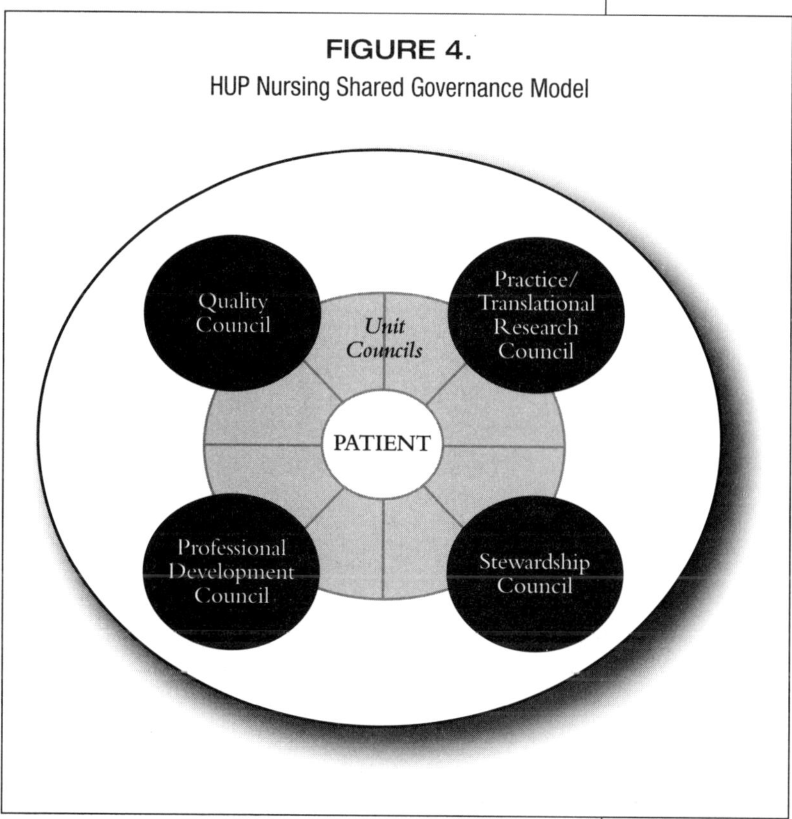

Perioperative Nursing

Between June 2005 and January 2006, HUP perioperative services faced several challenges in the nurse work environment that negatively affected nurse job satisfaction, as reported in the fall 2005 survey. The case volume had significantly increased, approximately 20% of the nursing staff had resigned and many of the remaining staff had 2 years of experience or less, and RN–MD and RN–RN relationships were strained. Not surprisingly, RN satisfaction had declined in several aspects of the Adapted Index of Work Satisfaction, though the scores remained in the moderate range (40 to 60).

Concerned with the declining satisfaction, the nursing leadership, with the support of hospital leadership and human resources, engaged the Center for Applied Research (CFAR) to address key process improvements to enable greater capacity and coordination, create a more respectful environment, enhance skilled communication, and empower clinical nurses through authentic leadership.

Through a retreat in early 2006 and using a technique known as backcasting, the CFAR team guided the HUP Perioperative Nursing Unit Council and other clinical nurses in addressing these challenges. The backcasting approach begins with specifying a goal or desired end state—envisioning an ideal future—and then proceeds to structured interviewing. Through the interview process, staff are guided in identifying obstacles to reaching the goal and identifying accomplishments to overcome the obstacles. A backcast map is developed that shows the obstacles and accomplishments. From this exercise, a project plan was developed (Hirschorn, 2007). The partnership of perioperative nurses and leadership established several task forces to address key issues contributing to dissatisfaction, including staffing and scheduling, education and orientation, and stress reduction. Each team developed a charter, a timeline, and an outline of key deliverables.

The staffing and scheduling task force recommended structure and process changes, such as the introduction of an evening resource pool and weekend premium program, and the addition of a leadership presence on the evening shift. The group also helped aggres-

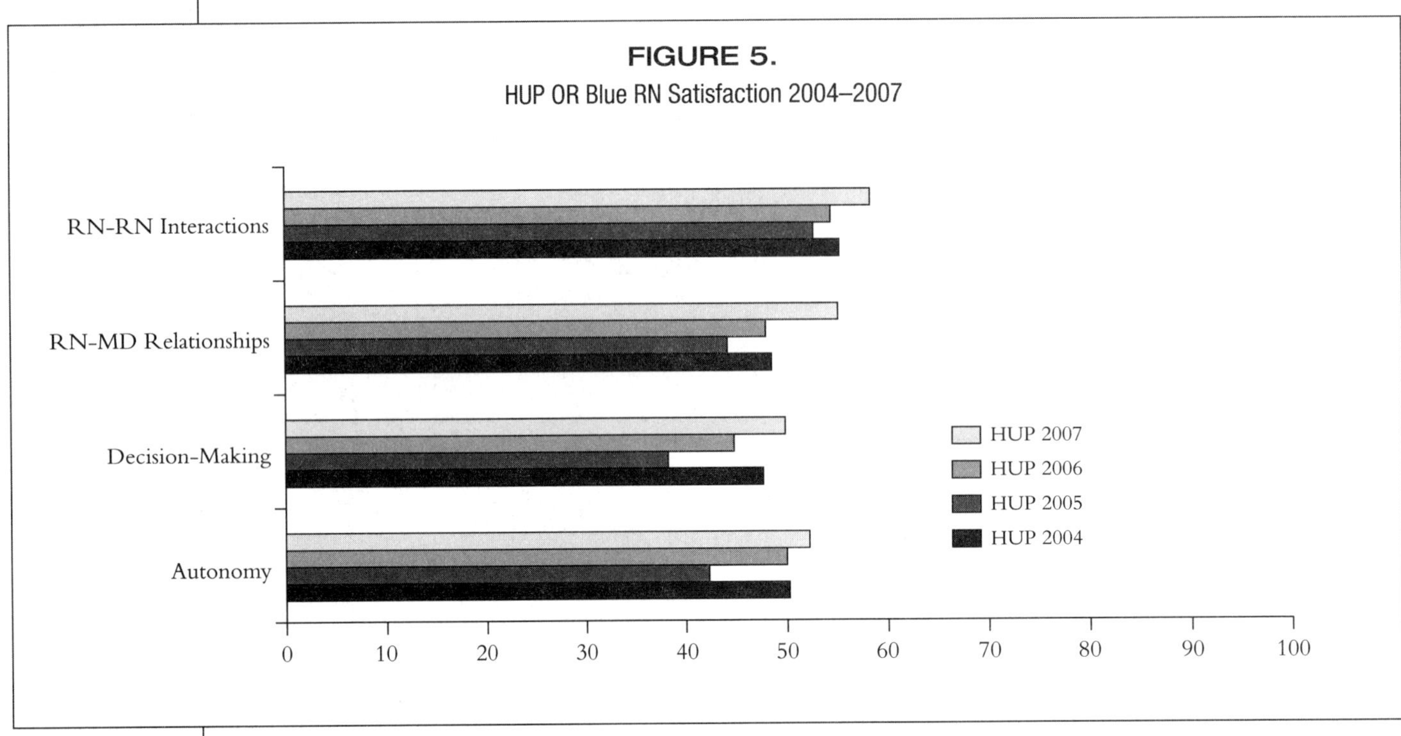

sively market the Gateway to Perioperative Nursing program (a robust orientation program for nurses new to perioperative nursing practice) and engaged clinical nurses in the interviewing process.

The education and orientation task force recommended modifying the Gateway program as well as extending the orientees' day-shift rotation and postponing the on-call requirement. This task force also obtained support for an additional full-time clinical educator.

The stress reduction task force recommended respectful workplace practices, adjustments to the relief shift, an overlapping shift from 11:00 a.m. to 7:30 p.m. that provided additional coverage and relief for lunch breaks, an increase in evening support staff, and assimilation of evidence-based practices and innovation, including improvements in instrument processing.

When faced with a decline in selected OR South RN satisfaction measures in 2005, the nurse manager reflected and then partnered with staff to strategize improvements. Together, they initiated an annual retreat day. The retreat was held on a Saturday to allow maximum participation, and staff were compensated for their time. The first retreat for clinical nurses and their care team partners (surgical technologists) included lectures based on identified learning needs, followed by a learning lab taught by clinical nurses for clinical nurses, in support of life-long learning. More recently, in 2007, the annual retreat learning lab included a team-building exercise that required team cooperation to win.

Clinical nurses in OR Blue also reported less satisfaction in 2005, compared with 2004, with RN–RN interactions, RN–MD relationships, decision-making, and autonomy. The nurse manager used the data as an opportunity to evaluate her process for daily assignments. Recognizing the importance of teamwork in the operating room and its relationship to patient safety, the clinical nurses now exercise autonomy and decision-making in determining the optimal team assignments (AORN 2008). Assignments based on work-style compatibility build trust and ensure a safety net in the operating room.

In response to declines in satisfaction related to RN–RN interactions and RN–MD interactions, the perioperative clinical nurses and their nurse manager in OR Blue include respect for others as an agenda item at all unit meetings. Nurses in the OR Blue unit, as well as clinical nurses across the hospital, are participating in "crucial conversations" training, modeled after the book by Patterson et al., to enhance skilled communication and strengthen team relationships (Patterson, Grenny, McMillan, & Switzler, 2002). A crucial conversation is a discussion between two or more people where stakes are high, opinions vary, and emotions run strong. The training supports nurses in learning the skills necessary to have difficult conversations in a constructive and respectful manner and promotes a healthy work environment.

It was also during this time frame that the Nursing Shared Governance model was developed and implemented. Early on, the transition from a manager-led governance structure to a shared governance structure involved learning new ways of working and interacting. In the early stages, councils focused on structure and process issues, such as staffing and scheduling, but have evolved to addressing outcomes and innovations in practice. The perioperative services have combined to form one unit council with clinical nurse members from each unit. The shared governance model has been effective in enhancing nurses' perceptions of decision-making and autonomy in the OR Blue unit, as reflected in their ratings of higher satisfaction with decision-making and autonomy in 2006 and 2007 (see Figure 5). Perioperative clinical nurses are eager for the opportunity to participate on the unit council and assume a formal leadership role that effectively influences their practice and work life.

As a result of these initiatives, not only have the OR Blue and OR South units noted improved RN satisfaction with the Adapted Index of Work Satisfaction and work contextual items, such as "Overall had a good day" (see Figures 6 and 7), they also have enjoyed a sustained decrease in the RN vacancy rate, from over 20% in 2006 to 0% in 2008. During the same period, agency use declined from five full-time employees (FTEs) to zero FTEs.

FIGURE 6.
HUP OR Blue RN Satisfaction—
Mean Values for Overall Had a Good Day 2004–2007

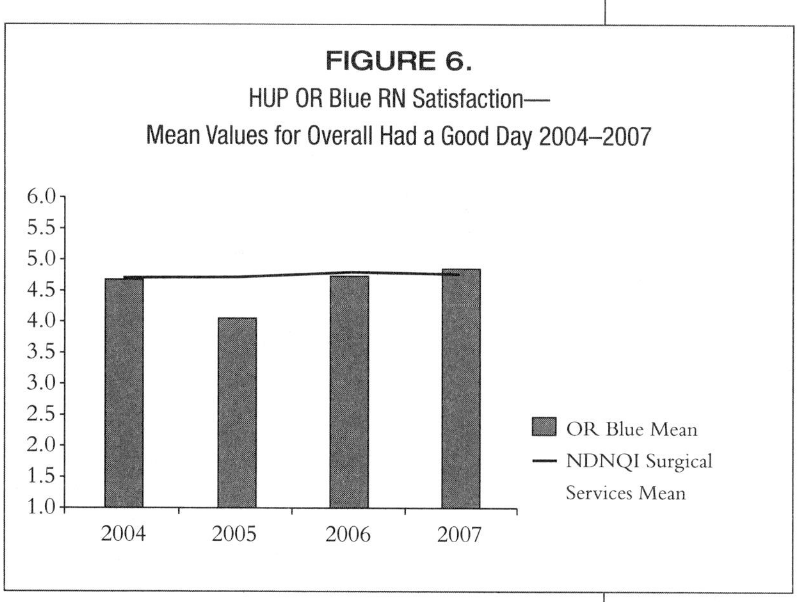

FIGURE 7.
HUP OR South RN Satisfaction Overall Had a Good Day 2004–2007

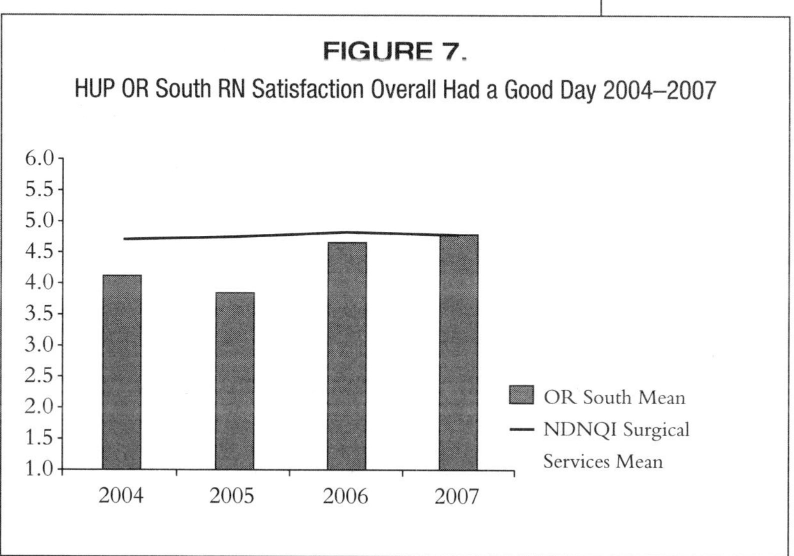

Emergency Department

The HUP Emergency Department processes approximately 59,000 visits a year. Over 30% of the hospital admissions are generated from the Emergency Department, primarily to medical units.

In 2005 and 2006, the Emergency Department RN satisfaction survey results demonstrated a decline from 2004 in satisfaction with task, decision-making, autonomy, job enjoyment, satisfaction with the status of nursing, and nurses' rating of the last shift: "Overall had a good day" (see Figures 8 and 9).

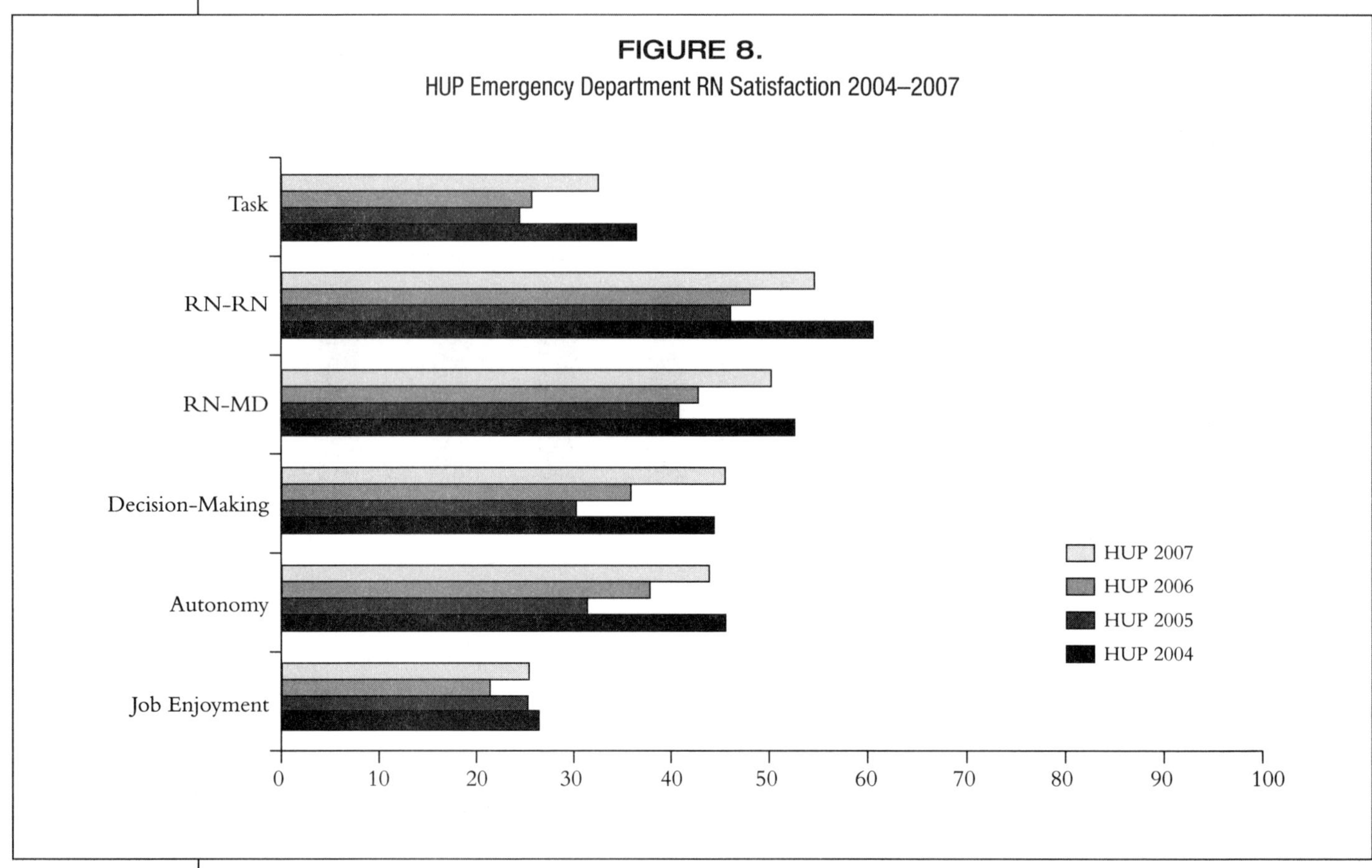

FIGURE 8.
HUP Emergency Department RN Satisfaction 2004–2007

Over these years, the Emergency Department had undergone significant changes in nursing leadership, and the clinical nurses, who reported to the ED physician chairman, were feeling isolated and disconnected from the hospital nursing department. Demonstrating authentic leadership, the chief nursing officer (CNO) intervened to provide leadership and stability. First, a positive working partnership was established with the physician chairman, and then an experienced interim clinical director was appointed. The interim clinical director was able to serve as a liaison between the Emergency Department and the hospital nursing department. Through meeting with the ED unit council and other clinical nurses, the CNO and clinical director partnered with clinical nurses in identifying key issues contributing to dissatisfaction, thereby decreasing the clinical nurses' sense of isolation. Initial efforts toward stabilization focused on structure and process aspects, including policies and procedures and scheduling. Additionally, a consultant was brought in to enhance team building within the ED staff, improve partnerships with physicians, and promote respectful communication. The ED clinical director, in partnership with a new and stable leadership team (nurse manager and clinical nurse specialist) and the unit council, was able to address concerns and implement improvements such as the following:

- Clearly define expectations for staffing, scheduling, and attendance
- Increase flex shifts
- Increase FTEs
- Enhance care team resources, such as pharmacy and respiratory services
- Boost supply and accessibility of equipment, such as stretchers and vital sign monitors

Once the foundational structures and processes were provided and the unit council was well established and fully functional, the ED team exercised autonomy and decision-making in enhancing their professional practice and development. Through the ED team's efforts, more nurses have oriented to the charge nurse, triage, and trauma roles, promoting role development and allowing greater flexibility in staffing. Clinical nurses have also engaged in teaching their peers, and more nurses have pursued clinical advancement and graduate education. Finally, the ED clinical nurses are participating on shared governance core councils and evidence-based practice groups, interfacing with nurses across the hospital and sharing their knowledge with the nursing community through professional presentations and publications and by participating in and leading community outreach programs. In response to staff concerns regarding safety, a security guard has been stationed in the unit and a metal detector has been installed.

By 2007, the ED clinical nurses were reporting satisfaction at or exceeding the 2004 baseline scores (see Figures 8 and 9). In addition, the ED RN vacancy rate decreased from 30% to 6%, while patient satisfaction scores increased in two areas: "Staff worked together to care for you," and "Likelihood of recommending the Emergency Department." Core measures improved for timely initiation of antibiotics for community-acquired pneumonia and the percentage of acute myocardial infarction patients who received aspirin on arrival. With an additional RN and certified nursing assistant (CNA) to staff the triage area, the "left without being seen" rate declined by 23%.

Given the initial success with the increased FTEs dedicated to triage, the clinical director was able to make a business case for additional RN FTEs over the next several years to support patient flow and to decrease waiting time. Other innovations in the planning stages are the establishment of POD assignments that group RNs, ED technicians, and physicians; development of waiting room guidelines; increased frequency of reassessments; the addition of a CNA to provide patient comfort measures and monitor vital signs; the reestablishment of a patient-flow nurse role; and revision of the diversion guidelines.

FIGURE 9.
HUP Emergency Department RN Satisfaction Mean Values Overall Had a Good Day 2004–2007

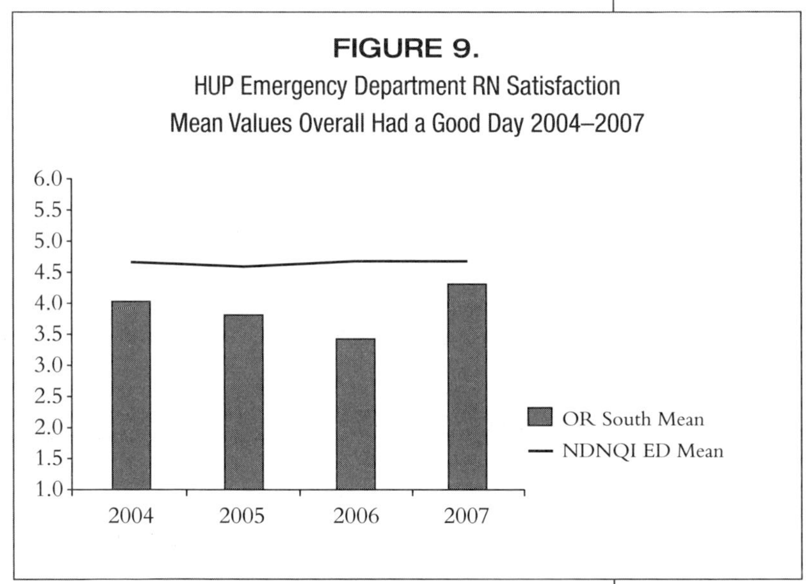

Clinical and Translational Research Center

The Clinical and Translational Research Center (CTRC), a National Institutes of Health (NIH)–sponsored unit within the Hospital of the University of Pennsylvania, has eight inpatient beds, three outpatient beds, and eight outpatient chairs. The unit cares for a variety of adult and elderly inpatient and outpatient research subjects. The unit has been staffed by a consistent group of clinical nurses with an average length of employment of 8 years. Thus, the clinical nurses and support staff have established positive working relationships with each other and with various researchers. Since beginning to participate in the RN satisfaction survey in 2004, the CTRC nurses have consistently reported high satisfaction (over 60) with task, RN–RN relationships, RN–MD interactions, professional status, professional development, nursing management, and job enjoyment (see Figure 10). In addition, they have responded positively to the item evaluation of last shift—"Overall had a good day" (see Figure 11).

FIGURE 10.
HUP CTRC RN Satisfaction 2004–2007

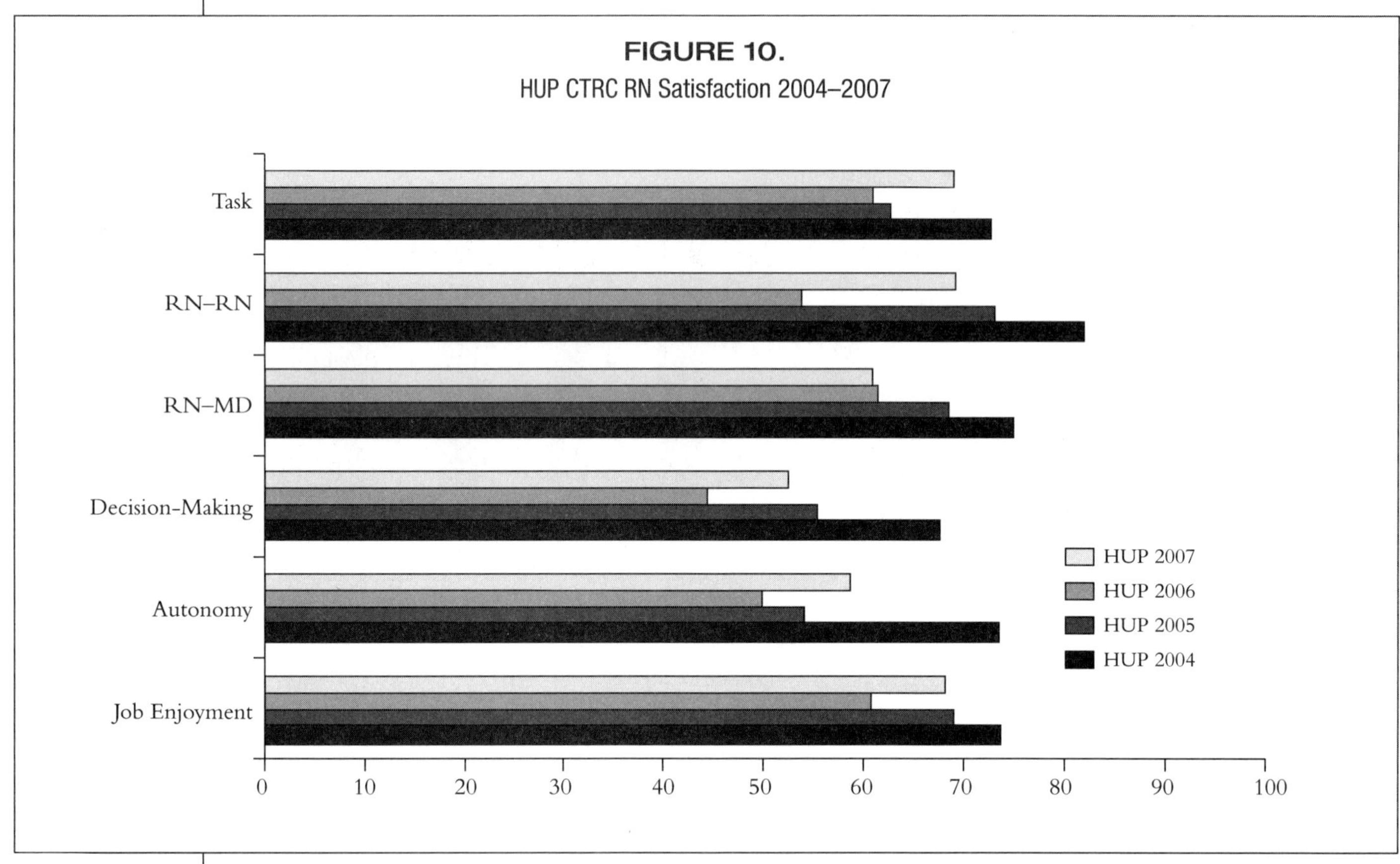

The unit clinical nurses and leadership attribute their sustained high satisfaction to a respectful environment, teamwork, continuing education regarding new studies, 1:1 nurse–patient ratio, and the manager's open-door policy. The clinical nurses report that they are reassured that their coworkers will support them and provide knowledgeable assistance whenever needed. They are knowledgeable regarding all active studies (up to 180 protocols at a time) and are respected by the researchers. The nurse manager is well known for having an open-door policy with her staff and all members of the healthcare team and strives to hear all concerns and facilitate problem-solving.

The clinical nurses reported moderate satisfaction with decision-making and autonomy in the early years of the RN satisfaction survey. Together, the nurse manager and unit council chair and members explored opportunities to enhance participation in the operation of the unit. Due to the nature of the research protocols, the nurse manager historically had managed the staffing and scheduling. The unit council identified this as an area in which they wanted more input. They instituted a self-scheduling committee and established self-scheduling guidelines. This change promoted satisfaction with flexibility and work–like balance, while meeting all of the needs of the unit and the study protocols. The Nursing Shared Governance framework provided opportunities for the CTRC nurses to participate in department-level committees and to address practice issues with clinical nurses across the unit. As result of these activities, a clinical nurse II was able to share her expertise and that of her colleagues with other nurses by developing a nursing policy on care of the human research subject. These opportunities contributed to sustained and improved ratings of satisfaction in many measures of the RN satisfaction survey in 2007 (see Figures 10 and 11).

Conclusions and Implications

Through a collective vision, HUP nursing leadership has transformed the culture of nursing practice over the past several years. The conceptualization of the professional practice model and the development of a shared governance model have enhanced the nursing work environment and related RN satisfaction feedback. Keys to success and positive changes include the following:

- The evolution of the satisfaction survey from a nurse manager–led process to a process guided by clinical nurse leaders in the role of unit council chairs.
- Demonstration of administration support and encouragement for clinical nurse participation in the survey by establishing incentive gifts for high response rates over the years.
- Shared accountability—among clinical nurses and nurse leaders—for action planning and implementation at the unit and department level.
- Clear evidence of the value of participation by sharing and highlighting initiatives generated as a result of RN satisfaction survey feedback over time.

FIGURE 11.

HUP CTRC RN Satisfaction Mean Values Overall Had a Good Day 2004–2007

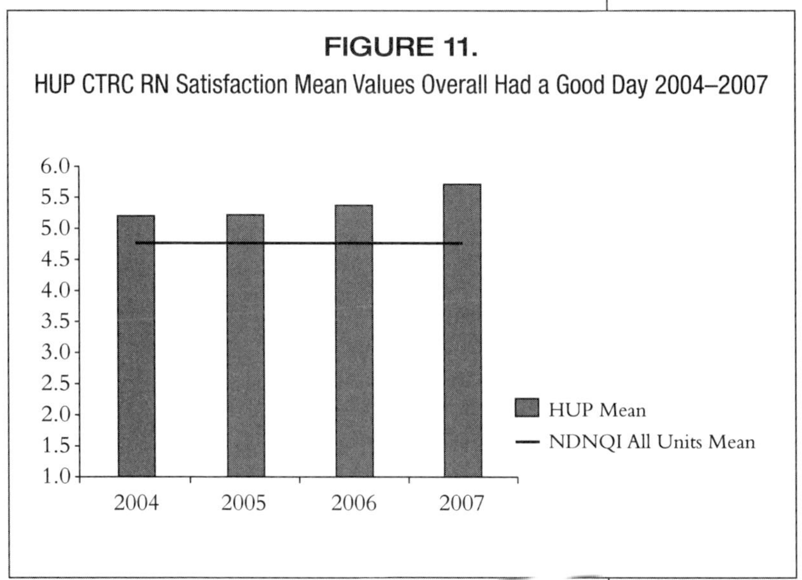

References

American Association of Critical Care Nurses (AACN). (2005). *Standards for Healthy Work Environments.* Aliso Viejo, CA.

Association of periOperative Registered Nurses (AORN). (2008). *AORN Position Statements: Statement on patient safety: Creating a patient safety culture.* Retrieved December 31, 2008 from http://aorn.org/PracticeResources/

Hirschorn, L. (2007). Backcasting a systematic method for creating a picture of the future and how to get there. *OD Practitioner,* 39 (4), 16–21.

Nursing Organization Alliance (NOA). (2004). *Principles and Elements of a Healthful Practice/Work Environment.* NOA: Lexington, KY

Patterson, K., Grenny, J., McMillan, R., & Switzler, A. (2002). *Crucial conversations: Tools for talking when stakes are high.* New York: McGraw Hill.

Using Best Practices to Improve RN Satisfaction

Becky Dodge, RN, MBA
Nursing Quality Analyst
bdodge@unch.unc.edu

Nimisha Patel, MHA
Coordinator, Magnet Program

Marilyn Pearson Morales, MSN, APRN, BC
Director, Nursing Practice, Education, and Research

Cathy Madigan, MSN, RN, CNAA-BC
Associate Chief Nursing Officer

University of North Carolina Hospitals

Editor's Pick

INSIGHTS & IDEAS FROM THIS FACILITY

Clinical nurse leaders, team-building activities, and shared governance, supported, unit-based initiatives to improve the nursing work environment. Example: Staff nurses being included on hiring committees

Facility and Unit Summary

FACILITY SUMMARY

Facility	University of North Carolina Hospitals—Chapel Hill, NC **www.unch.edu**
Facility setting	• Academic medical center, the state tertiary-care facility for the people of North Carolina • Full-service hospital, including Burn Center, Stroke Center, Level I Trauma Center, Level III Neonatal Intensive Care Unit, National Cancer Institute (NCI) Cancer Center
Teaching status	Academic medical center
Ownership status	Nonprofit, supported by the North Carolina state government
Community demographics	• Serves all 100 NC counties, with 80% of the patient population coming from 28 counties • Ethnicity: 56.7% white, 27.7% black, 7.4% Hispanic, 1% American Indian, 0.9% Asian, and 6.4% other • Approximately 11% of service area population over age 65
Hospital-staffed beds	720 staffed beds, 727 licensed beds
Case mix index (CMI)	1.52
Indicators used	Skin, Falls, Restraints, Nursing Staffing Information, Pediatric Peripheral IV, Pediatric Pain
System or unit improved	Pre-Care, Urology/Cystology (Uro/Cysto), Neurosurgery Intensive Care Unit (NSICU), Women's/Children's Post-Anesthesia Care Unit/Procedural Care Suites (PACU/PCS)
Indicators improved	RN Satisfaction: Decision-making; Intention To Remain On The Job
NDNQI® participation	Since 2004
Magnet™ status	"On the Journey"
Governance model	Shared governance structure
Awards and recognition	• Five specialties rank in the top 50 programs of their kind nationwide, 1 of 41 best in the United States • Leap Frog Hospital Quality and Safety Survey 2007 • Best Workplace Award for 2008, American Assembly for Men in Nursing

UNIT PROFILES

NSICU

Internal name	NSICU
Size and type	8-bed unit, trauma beds; neurosurgery intensive care
Staff summary	Average RN years on unit: 5; RN national board certification: 2 certified
Staff skill mix	26 full-time RNs, 2 part-time RNs, 2 clinical support technicians (CSTs) , 5 health unit coordinators
Nurse-patient ratio (NHPPD)	18.63 Total NHPPD
Organizational structure	One clinical manager, one assistant nurse manager

PRE-CARE

Internal name	Pre-Care
Size and type	Pre-operative screening area; 75–90 patients/day
Staff summary	Average RN years on unit: 4.5 years
Staff skill mix	10 RNs (2 master's-prepared), 4.5 medical support assistant IIs, x-ray tech, EKG tech
Nurse-patient ratio (NHPPD)	Not applicable
Organizational structure	One master's-prepared manager

URO/CYSTO

Internal name	Uro/Cysto
Size and type	5 rooms for procedures in OR; 12–25 patients/day
Staff summary	Average RN years on unit: 5.7; RNs are laser certified
Staff skill mix	6 RNs, 1 technician
Nurse-patient ratio (NHPPD)	1:1 for local anesthesia; 2 staff per patient for other procedures
Organizational structure	Charge nurse (CN-III)

WOMEN'S/CHILDREN'S PACU/PCS

Internal name	Women's/Children's PACU/PCS (Women's/Children's Post-Anesthesia Care Unit/Procedural Care Suites)
Size and type	• Women's Procedural Care Suites: 5 rooms • Women's PACU: 6 bays • Children's Procedural Care Suites: 7 rooms • Children's PACU: 6 bays
Staff summary	• Average RN years on unit: 4 years; certified manager
Staff skill mix	12 RNs in PACU, 6 in PCS, 3 unit secretaries, 4 nursing assistants
Nurse-patient ratio (NHPPD)	Per ASPAN Standards: Phase 1 (first 30 minutes)—1:1, remainder of recovery is 1:2
Organizational structure	Master's-prepared manager, Assistant manager, Charge nurse for each unit

Using Best Practices to Improve RN Satisfaction

Becky Dodge, RN, MBA
Nimisha Patel, MHA
Marilyn Pearson Morales, MSN, APRN, BC
Cathy Madigan, MSN, RN, CNAA-BC

University of North Carolina Hospitals

Introductory Summary

The University of North Carolina Hospitals (UNCH) is an academic medical center located in Chapel Hill, North Carolina. While UNCH provides services to the citizens of all 100 counties in North Carolina, 80% of the patient population is represented by the 28 neighboring counties. The Department of Nursing includes approximately 2,400 employees, of which 1,700 serve in the inpatient setting. UNCH is affiliated with the University of North Carolina School of Nursing. Twenty-six percent of the nursing team is younger than 30 years of age, with a mean age of 40. Ten percent of nurses are male, which is above the national average.

UNCH began participating in the NDNQI RN Satisfaction Survey in 2004. Currently, there are 52 units that participate in the survey. NDNQI acknowledged four UNCH units as "sustained improvers" on RN satisfaction performance scores in 2007. All of the units scored above the national average for their respective comparison groups. This article discusses the different strategies that each of the high-performing units employed to achieve their respective levels of RN satisfaction.

The following are common themes that emerged from the examination of the work environment in these four units:

- Effective leadership at manager and staff levels
- Staff-level participation in the nursing shared governance structure
- Effective communication and teamwork between the nurse manager and unit staff nurses

In addition to these four units, UNCH improved scores in all 11 categories of the NDNQI RN Satisfaction Survey. In 9 of the 11 categories, the hospital exceeded the 2007 national average. UNCH leaders and staff members believe the scores were positively influenced by a redesigned shared governance structure, maturation of the Clinical Ladder, and hospital-wide Commitment to Caring initiatives.

Background

In 2003, the nursing leadership team developed the Nursing Congress, a model of shared governance as a platform to engage staff in creative problem-solving to improve patient care. Monthly meetings gave Nursing Congress representatives the opportunity to bring their individual unit's successes and issues to the table. These meetings were led by two staff cochairs with mentorship provided by the associate chief nurse officer (ACNO). The initial shared governance model evolved, and in 2007 nursing adopted a new councilor model (see Figure 1). The steering com-

FIGURE 1.
Shared Governance Model

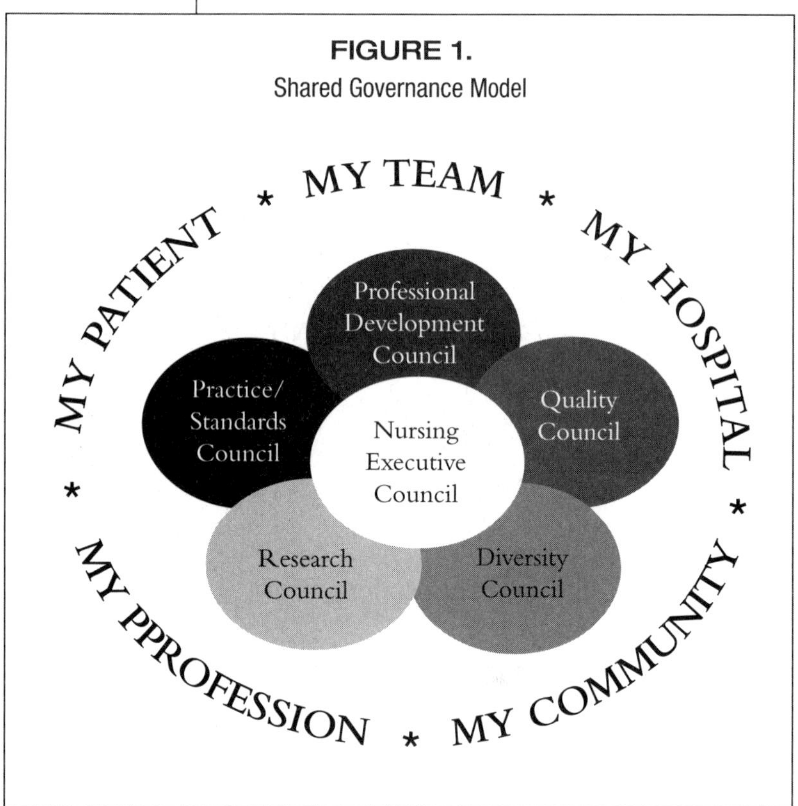

mittee for the new model—composed of one-third staff representatives (including two from the Nursing Congress), one-third managers, and one-third senior leadership—collaborated to design the new shared governance model. Direct input from staff RNs contributed to the success of the integrative structure that best represented the needs of the bedside nurse. By engaging staff in the developmental phase, nursing leadership demonstrated that they valued staff as equal partners and were committed to empowering nurses to participate in decision-making. The staff representatives also participated in the "go-live" process for the new shared governance model and continue to serve on the councils as cochairs or members.

The new shared governance structure comprises the following six councils:

- Professional Development Council
- Quality Council
- Diversity Council
- Research Council
- Practice/Standards Council
- Executive Council

Each council was led by a staff chair and cochair and met on a monthly basis. The Executive Council membership comprised the staff cochairs from each council, as well as the chief nursing officer (CNO), the two associate CNOs, and nursing directors. This model allowed greater emphasis on identified areas of nursing practice and a structured scope of responsibility for each council. Communication was bidirectional, with unit-level committees providing for the flow of information between councils.

The evolution of shared governance also included updating the mission, values, and philosophy statement, so that the goals and organizational culture were clearly communicated and represented. As a result, the Department of Nursing's mission is *to be a leader in providing compassionate, quality care focusing on the unique needs of patients and their families.* Additionally, core values for the department of nursing were created: *My patient, my team, my hospital, my community, and my profession.* Figure 2 shows the logo developed by the steering committee that represents these values. The logo is displayed on all nursing units and was developed into a button for nurses to wear on their name badges.

A Clinical Ladder, implemented in 2004, established a clear avenue for nursing staff career advancement. Based on Benner's (1984) Novice to Expert model, the clinical ladder defined four levels of clinical practice:

1. Clinical Nurse I (CN-I; novice)
2. Clinical Nurse II (CN-II; competent)
3. Clinical Nurse III (CN-III; proficient)
4. Clinical Nurse IV (CN-IV; expert)

To date, approximately 212 CN-IIIs and 71 CN-IVs

have been appointed. Many of these nurses have distinguished themselves by being active on UNCH councils and committees and by providing leadership support on their units.

In addition to these Department of Nursing initiatives, UNCH consulted with the Baptist Health Care Journey to Excellence and developed the Commitment to Caring campaign in spring 2007. The goal of Commitment to Caring at UNCH is to develop leadership that fosters a culture to achieve performance excellence. This program created goal congruence among every department in the hospital through a strategic framework focusing on six main components known as the *pillars*: people, service, quality, finance, growth, and innovation. The graphic representation of this framework (Figure 3) is easily recognizable by all hospital employees and reinforces the message of Commitment to Caring.

This framework has become common language among the UNCH team; meeting agendas and employee newsletters are organized according to these six areas, and decisions that influence patient care and hospital staff are aligned with the framework. On a daily basis, employees aim to fulfill the objectives of these six pillars. Eight different teams have been developed to guide the organization to meet each pillar's goal, and seven of the eight teams include nursing representation.

The *people* component directly relates to the employees of UNCH. Organizational initiatives, programs, and action items are implemented with the goal of creating a healthy work environment and highly satisfied employees.

Best Practices and RN Satisfaction in Four UNCH Units

Since NDNQI RN satisfaction reports are detailed by unit, four units in the nursing department at UNCH have been able to showcase their strengths. These units in particular scored above the national benchmarks, both overall and by specialty area: Pre-Care and Neurosurgery Intensive Care Unit (NSICU) for satisfaction with the survey's decision-making indicator and the Women's/Children's Post-Anesthesia Care Unit/Procedural Care Suites (PACU/PCS) and Uro/Cysto for the indicator "Intention to remain on the job." Leadership and staff are now examining these strengths and learning from these best practice areas to achieve even greater success for the entire nursing department.

FIGURE 2.
UNC Hospital Nursing Core Values

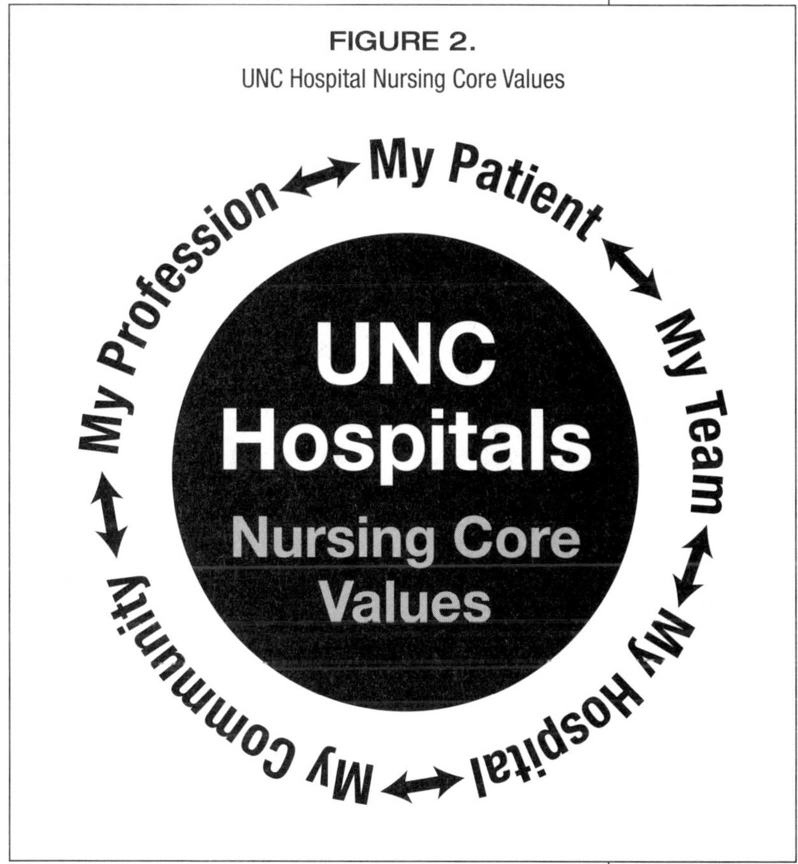

Pre-Care: Decision-Making

At UNCH, Pre-Care functions as the preoperative area where surgical patients receive perioperative education, nursing assessments, and anesthesia evaluation, or EKG, CXR, and laboratory services. The mission of Pre-Care is to promote operating room readiness by optimizing patient and chart preparation to avoid delays or risk of cancellation on the day of surgery.

FIGURE 3.
Commitment to Caring Pillars at UNC Hospitals

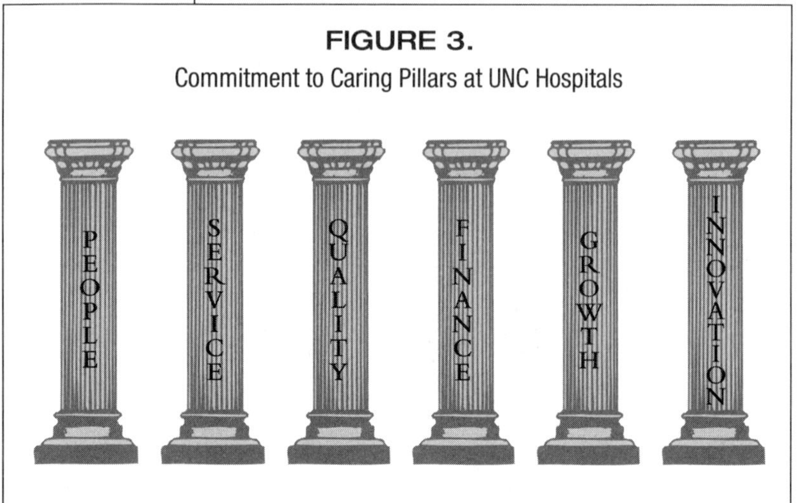

The Pre-Care nurse evaluates the preoperative workups that patients bring with them from the surgery clinic. The nurse also confirms the accuracy and completeness of patient information and ensures the patient has received all preoperative instructions.

Effective leadership

Prior to the current nursing manager, hired in 2000, there was high turnover of leadership at the unit level, with four managers in a 3-year period. With the lack of consistent leadership, inevitably the team became fairly dysfunctional and lack of trust existed among the staff.

The current nurse manager set out to develop a healthy work environment and collaborated with her staff to accomplish this goal. She provided the support needed in the unit to give staff the confidence to make decisions related to patient care. Staff began to feel empowered and became comfortable making choices that led to high-quality, safe patient care. Acknowledging the staff as individuals with varying ways of successfully accomplishing day-to-day tasks, the nurse manager provided them with autonomy to develop their own methods and solutions to deliver patient care. This gave the nursing team a sense of ownership for their work. As a result of this change in the work environment, the team felt empowered and autonomous, and trusted each other. This sense of teamwork allowed the further development of staff by rotating their assignments, including the role of charge nurse.

Empowerment

Staff members are encouraged to participate in the interview process as positions become open. This change allowed the current team and the candidates to spend time together discussing the roles and responsibilities of the job. At the conclusion of the interview process, participating staff provided feedback and made recommendations for candidate selection. This inclusion gave staff the opportunity to take ownership of this process and to select individuals with job-fit and team-fit characteristics, contributing to a strong sense of teamwork and accountability in the clinic.

Communication

Communication with physicians by the Pre-Care nursing staff often began with an apology for paging them to discuss a patient need and obtain or clarify an order. Guidance and mentorship by the nurse manager, regarding the importance of a nurse–physician collaboration as a critical success factor in providing the best possible care for each patient, changed this practice. Pre-Care nurses now communicate on a professional level with physicians and are considered by physicians to be valuable members of the interdisciplinary team.

Staff contribution to process changes

In 2006, the intake process for day surgery patients was changed. The nurses were involved in decision-making related to the new patient throughput process. Shift hours were changed to accommodate the new process and decrease the wait time for pre-operative patients. The nurses believed their input into these decisions made a difference in helping their patients get better care and also in using resources more effectively. This, in turn, positively affected nurse satisfaction.

Staff were also extensively involved in updating adult and pediatric preoperative information and education pamphlets. As content experts, nurses wrote and edited the information. They also wrote the scripts for the preoperative phone calls made to patients that were not able to have on-site pre-op teaching and assessment. Staff nurses continued the scripting process as they determined the best way to implement the new changes. Together they decided a dedicated RN would call this select group of patients, supplying them with clear and accurate information related to their procedure.

Implementing the shared governance model in the Pre-Care clinic resulted in five teams of nurses who make decisions on the projects that were undertaken. Some of the projects currently under way were focused on process improvement initiatives, educational offerings, competency validation, communication, and chart review/audits.

With the leadership of the current nurse manager and the ability of the unit nurses to embrace change, the Pre-Care team developed a positive, team-oriented approach in which individuals enjoy their work and feel empowered to provide safe, high-quality patient care.

Two consequences of these process changes have been decreased staff turnover and increased RN satisfaction with decision-making. Figure 4 shows the UNCH Pre-Care increase in scores from 2004 to 2007 compared with the national peri-Op NDNQI score. Data from the UNCH human resources department indicated that turnover decreased from a high of 20% in the first quarter of 2005 to 6.5% in the fourth quarter of 2007. Since 2006, the Pre-Care staff's satisfaction with decision-making has been among the top 25% of perioperative units participating in the RN survey, significantly above the NDNQI average.

FIGURE 4

Pre-Care Decision-Making Scores, 2005–2007

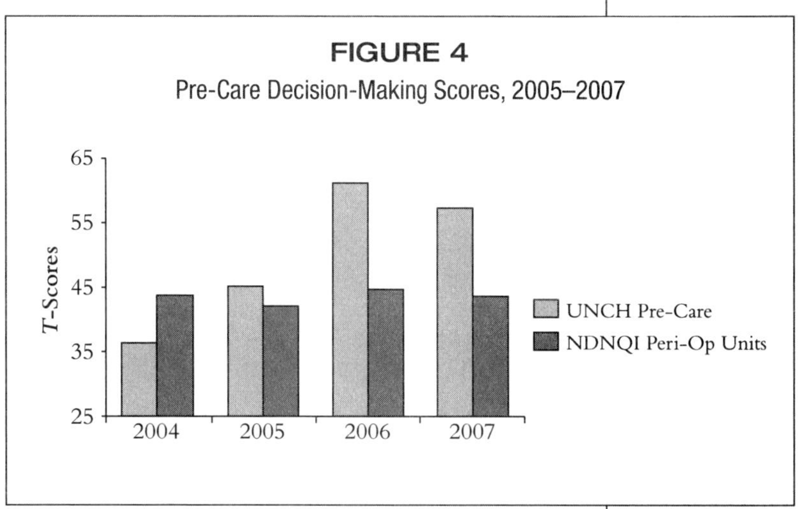

NSICU: Decision-Making

The Neurosurgery ICU (NSICU) is an 8-bed combined neurosurgery and trauma unit. New leadership began in October 2006, when the annualized turnover rate was at an all-time high. Many of the positive changes in decision-making began with the implementation of shared governance. Prior to this change, staff perceived that decisions were made by management, and staff were expected to meet the objectives of those decisions without any input. The culture began to change when staff were asked to identify issues and bring them to the unit's shared governance committee, thereby driving change through staff participation. In NSICU, every staff member is given the opportunity each quarter to serve on the unit committee. During their respective quarter, staff members communicate and identify any specific NSICU issues on behalf of the entire team to the unit's shared governance committee.

Staff contribution to process changes

Pyxis (medication) area. Staff expressed frustration with the clutter of supplies and disorganized nature of the area surrounding the pyxis. The first tangible initiative for the committee was to install a shelf over the pyxis area, with bins for improved organization. Though a small change, the systematic placement of materials greatly affected the staff's practice in a positive manner, since the pyxis was used numerous times during the nurse's shift. Being the first staff-led change, this resulted in excitement and appreciation for the new committee.

Bedside carts. Every patient's room has a cart stocked with frequently used supplies. Feedback from staff indicated that the carts were being stocked inadequately, they were disorganized, and items couldn't be easily located. As a solution, the staff participated in the evaluation of par lists to determine actual usage. The par list and number were adjusted to ensure consistency in stock. Drawer diagrams were also developed and posted on the carts so that all individuals stocking the cart referenced the same example for placement of supplies. This resulted in greater ease of locating items. Not only were staff satisfied with the improved bedside carts, they also believed that the organization and consistency of supplies led to better and more timely patient care.

Snack cart. Due to the fast-paced and complex nature of the unit, staff often don't choose to take time to leave the unit for breaks. As a result, the staff created a snack cart. The cart has easy access, as it is located in the middle of the unit, and staff can buy items for a modest price of 50 cents each. The snack cart has been such a success that staff from many different departments visit the NSICU to purchase items; some units have even reproduced the idea and created their own snack cart.

NSICU uses the revenue from the snack cart for reward and recognition. The following are two ways the money has been used:

- *T-shirts:* Staff decided to have NSICU T-shirts made. Staff recommended slogans and voted on the winner. Public Affairs and Marketing at UNCH created the design, and the T-shirts qualify as part of acceptable hospital dress code. T-shirts were purchased for every permanent staff member, creating visual unity.
- *Team activities:* Team-building activities have also added to increased staff satisfaction. As a side benefit to shared decision-making among staff, the NSICU team now has more involvement and camaraderie with each other. Quarterly off-campus activities were initiated to sustain the positive relationships between co-workers. The initial group activity was a trip to a local team baseball game. Everyone's ticket was paid for from the snack cart fund. To foster even more pride for the staff, one of the unit team members arranged for "Welcome NSICU" to be displayed on the scoreboard screen. The game was played in the evening, allowing day-shift staff to attend: in true team spirit the staff traded shifts with each other, and only five nurses from the night shift who wanted to attend weren't able to attend.

Development of CN-III leaders. As mentioned, previously, the Clinical Ladder implemented in the Department of Nursing provided a mechanism for career progression. The nurse manager, CN-IV, and CN-III are seen as the unit leaders and meet on a monthly basis to discuss unit operations. This type of meeting allows for both the CN-IV and CN-III nurses, who have applied and been approved for their role, to be exposed to day-to-day management issues that occur and to learn how to best deal with them. The CN-I and CN-II nurses, the health unit coordinators, and nursing assistants are assigned as a team to a CN-III leader. The designated CN-III leader helps mentor the team and provides pertinent education and information. While the CN-III is a unit leader, she or he is not in a management role. CN-I and CN-II staff view the CN-III as a peer and feel more comfortable approaching about questions or concerns. They take pride in knowing that they are being represented as staff when a CN-III is involved in the decision-making process. This process has helped to maintain the high decision-making scores.

All of the above examples have led to several positive outcomes:

1. The turnover rate is down to 10% according to internal Human Resources (HR) records.

2. Staff unity is apparent when entering the NSICU.

3. As seen in Figure 5, for the past 2 years the NSICU decision-making score far exceeds the NDNQI adult critical care average.

FIGURE 5.
NSICU Decision-Making Scores, 2004–2007

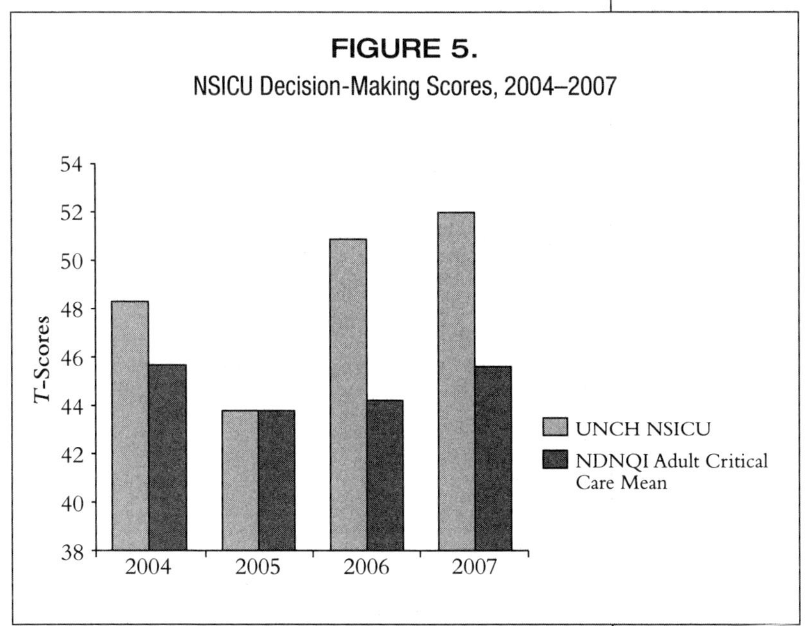

Women's and Children's Procedural Care Suites: Intention to Remain in Job

The Women's and Children's Post-Anesthesia Care Unit/Procedural Care Services is part of the comprehensive surgical services department at UNCH. The unit cares for 30 to 35 patients daily. Six PCS RNs and 12 PACU RNs collaborate to provide care to these patients. The RN staff is supported by three unit secretaries and four nursing assistants.

The unit leadership team's sustained effort to create a culture of teamwork, empowerment, and effective communication within their unit has been successful. The three components helped the department to retain RNs. Results from the NDNQI RN Satisfaction Survey report for the Women's and Children's PACU/PCS indicate 88% of RNs plan to remain in their job—higher than the 84% reported by nurses nationally. Also, the UNCH HR department reported that the unit's turnover decreased by 39% over the past 2 years, demonstrating the effectiveness of the improvements made to create an attractive work environment.

Prior to 2007, low nursing management visibility and reactive management approaches to common staff issues were the norm. The need to decrease turnover became a priority for the new leadership team when turnover peaked at 16.2% (internal HR measurement) in Q2-06. The unit leaders initiated several different processes for improving work culture, while engaging staff along the way, to determine what would work best for UNCH's Women's and Children's PACU/PCS.

Teamwork

When team members are not with patients, they meet around the nurse's station to collectively discuss the unit's workload and agree on how it will be accomplished. When the unit census is low, the nurses with no assigned patients assist the nurses who have patients. One of the nurses stated, "I not only see the nurse as my coworker, but as my friend, so I want to help whenever I can." The friendship dynamic stems from the social relationship that the nurses have outside the unit. The Women's and Children's PACU/PCS has a Sunshine Committee that is led by one of the staff nurses. The committee plans and organizes social events for the nurses outside of work, such as movie nights and self-care spa activities. Management encourages nonwork social activities, realizing the positive effect they have on the nursing team.

Empowerment

The leadership team in the PACU/PCS encourages the individual nurse to think analytically and creatively to develop a solution for identified problems. Nurses remedy their own challenges, but the leaders are always available for support or encouragement.

Effective communication

Team harmony and unity are facilitated with increased communication. First and foremost, the management team has an open-door policy, setting the tone for communication at any time and creating accessibility to managers. Being proactive about common staff issues eliminates built-up frustration that potentially can be carried over day after day. The absence of this frustration among staff contributes to a more positive work environment. The nurse managers consistently communicate and reinforce behavior expectations. Just as they see the value in applauding positive behavior, the unit leaders don't hesitate to immediately point out unacceptable behavior. Management recognizes that active listening is also part of a strong communication system. Staff state what they want to discuss in the monthly staff meetings, and those items are included on the agenda. For example, the Women's and Children's PACU/PCS team requested more interaction with the physicians, so the physicians were invited and attend staff meetings when possible.

Urology/Cystology Suites: Intention to Remain in Job

The nurses working in the Urology/Cystology suites have worked in the profession for 15 years or more. While turnover rates have not been high, there were issues that needed to be addressed in order to improve satisfaction among staff, ultimately leading to increased intentions to remain on the job. Figure 6 shows the progress made in this category from 2006 to 2007. This includes improving team-building and encouraging staff to take responsibility to make decisions on their own, to take responsibility for dealing with issues as they come up, and sometimes to have a "crucial conversation" with a coworker or other employee. The following ideas and interventions were implemented to build team unity and encourage individual initiative:

- *Educational presentations.* These were added to monthly staff meetings, and each staff member is designated to be a keynote speaker at a meeting. Staff members take turns presenting an interesting topic, an experience, or a class, promoting an atmosphere of shared learning and connecting with each other. When possible, staff attend CEU programs.
- *Autonomy.* At the monthly meetings, staff share stories about when they have independently resolved a problem encountered during the workday, thereby decreasing the number of times the charge nurse is called to intervene.
- *Communication.* One of the patterns in the unit had been for staff to come to the charge nurse when there was a conflict or issue that needed to be addressed. This behavior was not promoting professionalism or autonomy. Staff now resolve issues in a timely fashion, sometimes needing to be assertive and sincere at the same time with their actions and words. Staff are more aware of when colleagues are in need or overwhelmed. These changes allow team members to realize that they can resolve issues themselves, increase productivity, and promote a greater sense of respect among staff.

To improve trust and team-building, the staff performed an exercise that had been presented by a recent leadership development speaker. An obstacle course was laid out, a staff member was blindfolded, and a coworker guided the individual through the obstacle course. The exercise simulated the importance of teamwork, effective communication, and listening skills. It brought fun and laughter to the unit, and everyone who participated received a gift card for their bravery.

An additional exercise focused on communication and had everyone close their eyes and fold a piece of paper and rip corners off after voice commands. At the end of the exercise participants could see that, in spite of hearing the same commands, each paper was unique. The exercise highlights differences in processing thoughts even when the same information is communicated.

In summary, the newly established culture of increased staff participation, effective leadership development at the staff level, improved communication, and a greater sense of teamwork led to increased staff morale and a renewed sense of commitment to their unit.

Conclusions and Implications

The "high achiever" units have implemented innovative programs and ideas, with an emphasis on having staff-level decision-making. The overall goals of these initiatives are to create a strong team dynamic and an attractive, healthy work environment.

The individualized interventions for each unit resulted in increased satisfaction with decision-making on two units and higher intention to remain on the job in the other two units. The common themes identified in achieving these successes were effective leadership, staff engagement in process improvement initiatives, and improved communication and teamwork.

Further, organization-wide changes have taken the nursing department as a whole to a higher level of nurse satisfaction. Since 2004, the Department of Nursing made improvements in every category on the NDNQI RN Satisfaction Survey. In 2007, RNs in UNCH units reported significantly higher levels of satisfaction than RNs in NDNQI national comparison units in task, RN–RN interactions, decision-making, pay, and nurse management.

A major benefit of combining staff-driven change with increased leadership at the unit level is a culture of empowerment, autonomy, teamwork, and professional development that is sustainable over time, leading to increased RN satisfaction.

UNCH's individual unit successes really showcase the diverse strengths across the entire department. The goal is to achieve similar successes on every unit in the nursing department. One way UNCH will accomplish pervasive, high RN satisfaction is by continuing the momentum of nursing leadership at the unit level by increasing the number of employed CN-IIIs and CN-IVs. To this end, the organization recently held their inaugural Aspiring Nurse Leader's Week, organized by the Professional Development Council. It was well received by the entire organization. This celebration included a keynote speaker and numerous continuing education opportunities for staff centering on leadership development. Also, since the Department of Nursing has exemplar units with high RN satisfaction, they have been able to identify key characteristics nurse managers and nurses have that set the stage for a healthy work environment. When hiring new members of the nursing team, they aim to recruit individuals who embody these characteristics. This method is part of a larger organization initiative termed Hiring for Excellence, which helps managers hire and retain people that are the right fit for the right position.

FIGURE 6.
Uro/Cysto Intention to Remain in Job, 2006–2007

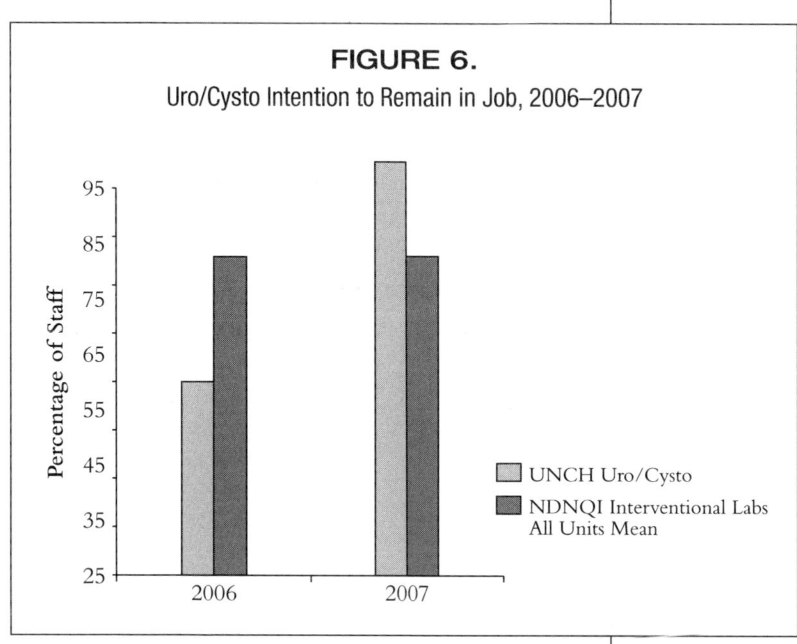

With all of the recent initiatives combined from the organizational level with Commitment to Caring and at the nursing department level with the new shared governance model, UNCH is able to engage a greater number of staff by giving them a platform to discuss issues as a team and develop solutions to improve nursing practice. The Department of Nursing intends to continue this type of collective thinking and increased autonomy and decision-making by hardwiring these initiatives. On the horizon, UNCH will integrate a nursing practice care-delivery model, Relationship-Based Care, into the existing frameworks.

All efforts to solidify a highly satisfactory work environment for nurses assists UNCH to meet its strategic goals for growth. With the new cancer hospital slated to open in the summer of 2009, as well as other new developments, there will be openings for nursing professionals, and an attractive work environment will draw nurses to be part of the UNCH nursing team.

References

Benner, P. (1984). *From novice to expert: Excellence and power in clinical nursing practice.* Menlo Park: Addison-Wesley.

Improving RNs' Rating of "Overall Had a Good Day"

Tammy Daniel, RN, BSN, CCRN, MHA
Assistant Administrator, Nursing
tammy.daniel@bmcjax.com

Tracey Johnson, RN, BSN
Director Surgical Services

Lucinda Deputy, RN, BSN, NA-BC
Director Women's Services and Intensive Care

Michele Causey, RN, BSN
Nurse Manager 3B MSP Medical–Surgical Unit

Christine Johnson
Director Human Resources

Baptist Medical Center South—Jacksonville, Florida

Editor's Pick

INSIGHTS & IDEAS FROM THIS FACILITY

Surgical services team conducted survey to identify needed changes in work environment. When implemented, RN satisfaction improved.

Facility and Unit Profile

FACILITY SUMMARY

Facility	Baptist Medical Center South (BMCS)—Jacksonville, FL **http://community.e-baptisthealth.com/bmc/south/**
Facility setting	BMCS, a 248,000-sq-ft, hospital with 120 suites on a 32-acre campus, is a full-service healthcare facility whose services include radiology, surgery, emergency services, oncology, and a sleep lab
Teaching status	Nonteaching hospital
Ownership status	Community based
Community demographics	Service area is primarily southern Duval and northern St. Johns counties, Florida, which includes Jacksonville and St. Augustine, with 80% of the patient population coming from 28 counties • Ethnicity 56.7% white, 27.7% black, 7.4% Hispanic, American Indian, 0.9% Asian, and 6.4% other • Approximately 1.4% of service area population over age 65
Hospital-staffed beds	120 staffed beds
Case mix index (CMI)	1.98
Indicators used	RN Satisfaction: Overall Had A Good Day
System or indicator improved	3B MSP (Medical-Surgical-Progressive) and Surgical Services
Indicator improved	RN Satisfaction: Overall Had a Good Day
QI report document used	FAST Methodology
NDNQI® participation	Since 2005
Time frame of QI experience	2005–2007
Magnet™ status	Magnet designation, December 2007
Governance model	Unit councils meet in a shared governance group

Awards and recognition	• HealthGrades Distinguished Hospital Award for Clinical Excellence: 100 Best Places to Work in Healthcare—2008 • Best Hospital in Northeast Florida in Folio Weekly's "Best of Jax" issue—2008 • U.S. News & World Report's Best Hospitals—2007 • Jacksonville Magazine named Baptist Health among its • "25 Companies That Care"—2004, 2005, 2006, 2007 • Cerner Leo Black Award for Innovation in Information Technology (to Baptist Health)—2005 • Florida Medical Business readers "Golden Stethoscope Award" for Best Use of Technology in Hospital or Health System—2006 • JEA IP Environmental Stewardship Award—2006 • Excellence in Employee Development Award, University of North Florida—2005
Staff summary	235 full-time RNs, 63 part-time RNs
Organizational structure	Chief nursing officer, Nursing directors, Assistant nursing administrator, Nurse managers

UNIT PROFILES

3B MSP

Internal name	3B MSP (Medical-Surgical-Progressive)
Size and type	24 beds; combined labor and delivery, recovery, and post-partum unit.
Staff skill mix	• NHPPD: 10.42 • RN total hours: 76.9 • Nurse–patient ratio: Day—1:5; Night—1:5–6 • RN education: Diploma, 6%; ADN, 41%, BSN, 39%; MS or PhD, 10%

Surgical Services

Internal name	Surgical Services
Size and type	6 OR Suites, 1 Cysto suite, 18 ASU rooms, 12 PACU bays
Staff skill mix	• NHPPD: N/A • RN total hours: 77.6 (total paid FTEs) • Nurse–patient ratio:OR and PACU, 1:1; ASU, 1:6 • RN education: ADN, 64%; BSN, 32%; MS or PhD, 4%

Improving RNs' Rating of "Overall Had a Good Day"

Tammy Daniel, RN, BSN, CCRN, MHA
Tracey Johnson, RN, BSN
Lucinda Deputy, RN BSN NA-BC
Michele Causey, RN, BSN
Christine Johnson

Baptist Medical Center South—Jacksonville, Florida

Introductory Summary

Baptist Medical Center South (BMCS), which opened February 16, 2005, is Jacksonville's first hospital of the 21st century and is the first newly constructed hospital to open in the area in over 20 years. Baptist Health's knowledge of the local market, combined with its planning process, identified the Southside of Jacksonville and northern St. Johns County as an area where additional hospital capacity was needed to address the area's increasing demand for health care. Given the area residents' historical utilization of BMC-Downtown (BMCD), the new hospital would also allow area residents to receive healthcare services in the community where they live rather than having to travel to BMCD, acknowledging the significant residential development in the area, which further increased the need for a hospital within the community.

The 254,000-square-foot BMCS opened with 92 acute care beds that are housed in three 24-bed medical/surgical nursing units, a 12-bed intensive care unit, 18-bed day stay unit, and 12 maternity suites. The hospital provides extensive outpatient diagnostic and testing services along with an 18-room emergency department. The hospital currently has 488 physicians on staff. In December 2006, BMCS received accreditation as a Primary Stroke Center through the Joint Commission. As of February 2007, BMCS has a bed capacity of 120 beds and plans to add an additional patient tower to meet the growing needs of the patient population.

Baptist Health is a five-hospital system located in Jacksonville, Florida, with Baptist Medical Center South as a part of this system. Baptist Health is a faith-based, mission-driven, locally governed organization dedicated to providing high-quality care for everyone. When BMCS opened in February 2005, Baptist Health nursing leadership had decided to apply for Magnet™ designation and determined that the National Database for Nursing Quality Indicators (NDNQI®) would be used for collecting nursing-sensitive quality indicators.

Baptist Health recognized that a new hospital provided a "greenfield" opportunity, one where the health system could look at developing innovative approaches to hospital operations rather than maintaining the status quo. Two of the most significant of these developments at Baptist South are the completely digital, or "paperless," environment in which the hospital operates and the environment for healing in which patients and their families recuperate and recover. While seemingly very different, these two accomplishments work together to improve patient outcomes.

Baptist Medical Center South: "The Digital Hospital"

The goal to open BMCS as a purely digital hospital was set early in the hospital's development by Baptist Health's chief executive officer and members of executive management. The team realized how difficult it would be to eliminate paper medical records and processes from the hospital if paper was ever introduced. More important, the leadership team recognized that electronic systems would provide tools to improve outcomes and enhance patient safety. The systems would provide caregivers with the latest and most accurate medical information for making treatment decisions. The system would also enhance patient safety by minimizing the common pitfalls associated with handwriting and abbreviations, as well as provide automatic allergy and drug dosage alerts. The planning process to open BMCS as a digital hospital was initiated in September 2003 and achieved the digital goal when the hospital opened in February 2005. The scope of the information systems within the digital hospital includes the following:

- Computerized physician order entry (CPOE)
- Physician documentation and electronic signature
- Nursing and ancillary documentation
- Automation of emergency department (triage and tracking, discharge instructions, prescription writer, ED physician documentation), surgery, laboratory, radiology/imaging, labor/delivery/recovery/postpartum, health information management (HIM), and scheduling
- Maternal and newborn documentation
- Materials management inventory and replenishment
- Filmless radiology and online EKG

The medical staff bylaws at BMCS required that physicians use the electronic system as a condition to practice at the hospital. In exchange for this commitment, Baptist Health devoted significant resources to make sure that support was available to any clinician who needed help with the new system. It was also important for the hospital to have an ample number of computers for all physicians and staff to be able to simultaneously access the system. The hospital provides multiple computer options to ensure access, including stationary desktop computers, mobile computers on wheels, and portable tablet PCs that connect to a hospital-wide wireless network, including the medical office building. In addition, physicians can securely access the system from their offices and homes. BMCS's digital environment has garnered much attention nationally, including a *Computerworld* cover story proclaiming "The Paperless Office—Really! How BMCS built an all-electronic environment while bigger, more prestigious hospitals failed." In addition, Baptist Health was featured in Intel's article "Unlocking Medical Information," which highlights the partnership between Intel and Baptist Health and the use of Intel's mobile technologies as being the key to digital success at Baptist Health.

NDNQI Participation, Part of the Magnet Journey

The Baptist Health philosophy for professional nurses is to provide the highest quality of nursing care to the patient, not only as an individual, but also as a member of the community. The belief that all nurses have the ability to promote excellence and leadership is demonstrated daily in nursing decisions and practice. On the basis of this philosophy, Baptist Health began participating in the NDNQI RN Satisfaction Survey in 2005.

As a commitment to this philosophy, Baptist Health made the decision to apply for Magnet recognition through the American Nurses Credentialing Center (ANCC). A necessary component was a scientifically validated process to measure nursing and patient outcomes as well as reliable comparisons of nursing-sensitive quality measures. BMCS committed to include nursing staff as much as possible in the data collection and to promote evidence-based practice that would provide the framework for clinical interventions. The

NDNQI provided unit-level performance reports that included comparisons with other units of the same type in same-size hospitals.

The RN Satisfaction Survey, a nursing measure available in NDNQI, enabled the staff to collectively verbalize their feelings and concerns related to nursing practice at BMCS. As with any survey, the staff were concerned about confidentiality. Confidentiality was maintained based on NDNQI's data collection and reporting practices. The Internet-based survey enabled the RNs to complete the survey at work or from home. Managers supported completion of the survey by providing patient care coverage as needed.

Ever since opening, Baptist Medical Center South committed to a flat organizational structure. Assistant nurse managers (ANMs) managed service lines and reported to service line nursing directors. Nursing directors reported to the assistant administrator of nursing who in turn reported to the administrator. The structure was absent nurse managers and ANM coverage for each nursing unit. ANMs were acting as charge nurses, managing shifts along with their patient assignments.

Senior leadership at BMCS saw a need for an increased management presence and began to hire additional ANMs for each nursing unit in late 2005. The nursing staff responded positively to the increased presence of ANMs as resources. In 2006 and into 2007, many ANMs began to assume additional administrative roles and provide even more extensive management support while allowing the nursing directors to focus on global issues in the facility. There is believed to be a positive correlation between the additional management presence and increased nursing satisfaction as evidenced in the NDNQI scores for 3B MSP and Surgical Services.

Many factors become evident when opening a fully electronic new hospital in a rapidly growing area. The initial volume for BMCS was grossly underestimated. Therefore, all staff became resilient and cohesive. While orienting to a new, completely electronic environment, the staff were also faced with an increased patient load, dwindling supplies, and understaffing. While senior leadership worked diligently to provide the necessary resources, all bedside staff worked to provide quality care to patients in less than optimal conditions. From that bonding and resilience flourished a culture of caring that still exists today.

A System for Supporting Nurturing Excellence

A high priority for the BMCS nursing leadership was to ensure that a practice environment of excellence was in place to support high-quality nursing practice and thus high-quality care for patients and their families. The shared leadership structure (Figure 1) was used to change the practice environment by enhancing communication, autonomy, education, and appreciation.

Communication

BMCS was one of the first facilities within Baptist Health to provide e-mail accounts to all employees as a means of internal communication. In addition to monthly staff meetings, e-mail is widely used to communicate daily with all staff. In fact, at BMCS it is expected that all employees will read and respond to e-mail. It has become second nature for the BMCS staff and leadership to rely on e-mail for process changes, additions, and daily "need to know" information. It is not unusual for staff to receive an e-mail from members of senior leadership within BMCS as well as from the Baptist Health system office. This provides a hands-on feeling of acceptance and appreciation for all staff. The chief nursing officer (CNO) publishes the "CNO Newsletter" for nursing leaders with the expectation that it will be forwarded to all employees and provided in hard-copy on each nursing unit. This gesture further cements the open communication pattern that senior leadership at Baptist Health expects and upholds.

FIGURE 1.
The BMCS Shared Leadership Structure

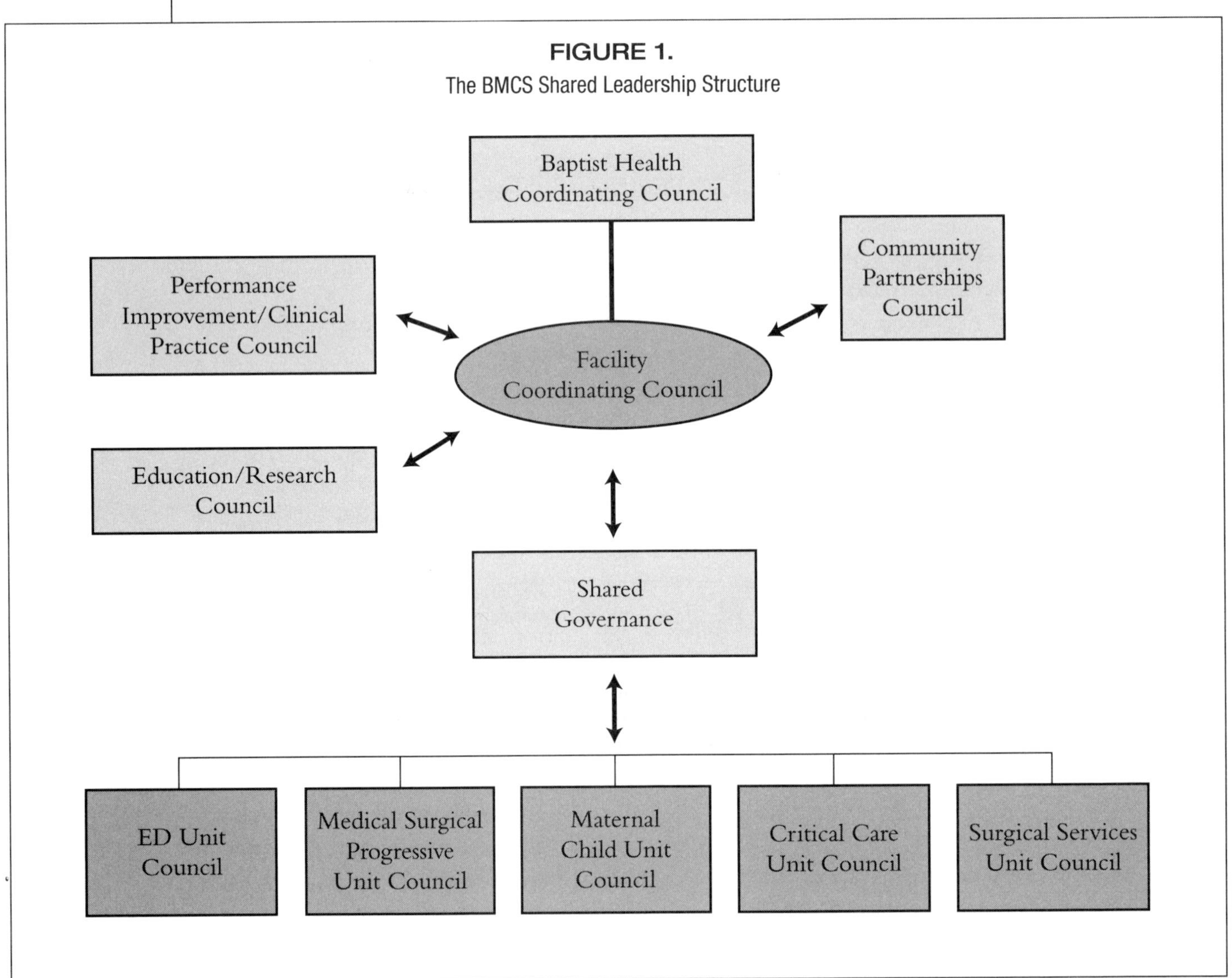

Communication at BMCS is also supported and encouraged through quarterly employee forums. Employee forums consist of one or two representatives from each department, along with the entire administrative team. Lunch is provided for employees to enjoy while leadership representatives present a program on the five critical success factors: people, service, quality, finance, and growth. The process then takes on a town hall forum process, as each unit representative brings forth questions on behalf of colleagues. The representative then relays answers and information to the unit staff. This process has fostered open communication with senior leadership and gathered answers to questions that staff may have.

Shared governance within Baptist Health is fostered by Magnet standards. Unit councils were formed on units as change catalysts, with the presumption that all practice changes should begin at the bedside with direct care providers. Monthly council meetings are held on each unit, and changes are advanced to unit management. For process and practice changes, council requests are brought to the Shared Governance Group, which comprises all unit council chairs. A shared governance chair is voted in by his or colleagues. Each unit council chair brings forth individual unit issues, and a vote is taken. The shared governance chair brings issues to the Facility Coordinating Council (FCC). The FCC is chaired by the facility's nurse executive and comprises facility managers, directors, and department heads. Issues approved by the FCC are brought to the system-level group of nurse executives from each facility, which is chaired by the chief nursing officer. Approvals and modifications are then sent back down to staff through their unit management. The unit council structure provides autonomy and empowers staff to own their practice and be accountable for patient outcomes as well as professional outcomes.

Nursing Autonomy and the ExCEL Model

Autonomy is nurtured through the Excellence in Clinical Education and Leadership (ExCEL) model (Figure 2), which is a Baptist Health professional development program designed to enable participants to select and pursue opportunities to meet their professional aspirations in nursing. The program recognizes and rewards the accountability of registered nurses in pursuing opportunities for advancing education and clinical expertise in their nursing field.

The ExCEL program is based on Benner's research that delineated five levels of expertise in nursing practice based on experiential learning (Benner, 1984). The five levels include the novice, advanced beginner, competent, proficient, and expert nurse. The levels are distinguished by the nurse's ability to independently implement the nursing process and individualize the plan of care based on patient or population needs.

Education

Baptist Health promotes and supports education for all staff throughout its facilities. In-house education is abundant throughout the system for all mandatory topics, including adult, pediatric, and neonatal care, and basic and advanced life support. Skill advancement opportunities are also offered in-house, including cardiac monitoring and interpretation. Baptist Health's employee home page provides information on educational opportunities for employees, including

FIGURE 2.

The Four Domains of ExCEL
(Excellence in Clinical Education and Leadership)

I. Professional Development and Citizenship

- Hospital Committee Participation
- Community Volunteer
- Community Health and Wellness Education
- National Nursing Certifications
- University Class Enrollment
- Presentation to Professional Group
- Special Projects
- Participation on a Clinically Relevant, City-Wide Committee or Task Force
- Employee Health/Wellness Education
- Internal certifications
- System Nursing Experience
- Self-Study Module
- Patient/Staff Educational Materials

II. Leadership and Service Excellence

- Committee Chairperson or Cochair
- Member of Nursing Organization
- Instructor certification
- Nursing In-service Presentation or Coordination
- Facilitation of a Support Group
- Unit Project Demonstrating Leadership, Teamwork, and Motivation
- Medical Record/Chart Review/Chart Audits/Peer Review
- National Patient Safety Goal Surveillance Projects

III. Evidence-Based Practice and Clinical Nursing Research

- Patient Care Intervention/Case Study
- Lead/Co-Lead Clinical Research Journal Club
- Data Collection for Nursing Research
- Attendance EBP/Research Workshops
- Attendance Nursing Research Journal Club
- Article Writing
- Membership Clinical Practice Council
- Participation on Clinical Practice Council
- Grant Writing
- Research Council Membership
- Research Council Participation
- International Nursing Caring Database
- Best Practice Identification
- Nursing Peer Review Committee
- Patient Care Problem/Issue

IV. Clinical Technology and Innovation

- Introduction to Technology
- Education
- Technological Research
- Technology/Tools Equipment Validation

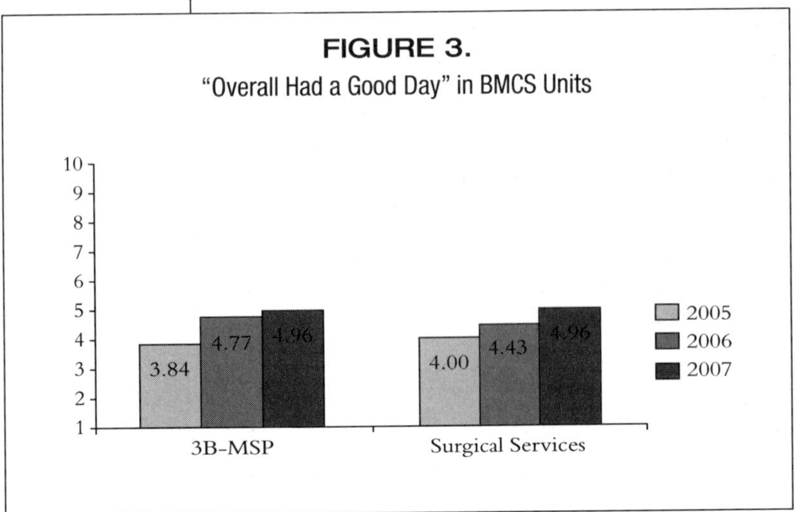

FIGURE 3.
"Overall Had a Good Day" in BMCS Units

e-learning. An in-house electronic system is available for registering, completing, and tracking educational opportunities.

Baptist Health teams with local universities to offer RN-to-BSN and RN–MSN programs. Tuition reimbursement is provided through the Learning and Educational Assistance Program (LEAP). After a staff member's initial probationary period, she or he is eligible for $2,000 per year for undergraduate work, $3,000 per year for graduate studies, $1,200 per year for certification and recertifications, and $500 per year for courses.

The Emerging Leaders program is a 1-year educational process designed to build the leadership skills of high-potential, nonmanagement employees. Based on admission criteria and acceptance, participants demonstrate the internal leadership qualities defined in the Baptist Health ExCEL model: integrity, self-awareness, self-discipline, compassion, insight, and courage. Over the course of the year, participants build fundamental management skills. They have an opportunity to demonstrate these skills on project teams and committees. Upon program completion, employees have the necessary skills and project experience for an entry-level supervisory position.

Appreciation

BMCS has a foundational belief in recognizing employees for their efforts. Each nursing unit is provided budgeted resources to recognize employees. Nursing leaders receive recognition toolkits complete with stars, note cards, movie tickets, and innovative suggestions for use. Employees receive individual handwritten notes from their leadership, candies and chocolates, dessert cards, movie tickets, and other personal trinkets. Pizza parties can be given by leadership for unit recognition. The Shining Star program allows coworkers to recognize each other with monthly submissions that are judged by a panel. Shining Star recipients receive a personal award presentation by the entire administrative team along with their picture on the Wall of Fame and a designated parking space for a month.

Recognition of all service by staff is an important part of the BMCS culture and an expectation for management.

Improvement in "Overall Had a Good Day"

The two units at BMCS showed sustained improvement on the "Overall Had a Good Day" question. They represent two different practice domains. (See Figure 3.)

3B MSP Care

The Medical-Surgical-Progressive (3B MSP) unit had to accommodate frequent overflow from Labor and Delivery, Recovery, and Post-Partum (LDRP). This posed many challenges for the nursing staff because of the change in patient population. Having mothers and babies on 3B MSP posed logistical challenges for the staff. While 3B MSP provided family-centered care to patients and their families, security for mothers and babies on overflow to 3B MSP required locked doors, increased security awareness, cameras, and doorbells.

Further, 3B MSP had to accommodate additional LDRP staff. The MSP staff learned to work in the enhanced security environment and incorporated the additional safety and security measures into practice.

At its inception, the LDRP Unit Council included staff members from 3B MSP. As a group, they brainstormed to resolve issues related to the overflow of LDRP patients and its impact on 3B MSP. The unit council asked for security cameras to be placed at both entrances to 3B MSP and played a large part in the ideal placement of additional supplies, telephones, and computers to ensure that the nursing staff had optimal work space. In the beginning, using in-house education resources, there was a group effort to cross-train the medical/surgical nurses in post-partum care so that they could manage the overflow assignments. Some nurses discovered their interest in caring for mothers and babies and subsequently transferred to the LDRP unit.

Surgical Services Unit

Baptist Health uses the FAST methodology (Figure 4) to facilitate performance improvement teams:

F—Focus on specific aim
A—Analyze basic data
S—Select potential changes
T—Test potential changes

Focus

A focus statement can be developed by specifying an aim for the improvement project and setting a numerical target for this improvement. "To improve patient satisfaction related to Outpatient Procedures Goal: To improve Gallup scores to 90%."

Analysis

Team discussion led to analysis of the outpatient surgery flow process and the identification of possible dissatisfiers or bottlenecks for patients, caregivers, staff, physicians, and volunteers. A team was identified to ensure that a sufficient diversity of perspectives was represented to identify issues; however, all staff were invited to attend the meetings, which were scheduled in the afternoon, after cases were completed. To ensure that all surgical staff could give input, an electronic survey was developed based on issues identified in the meetings. The survey was conducted twice in order to identify and confirm issues. Information from team meetings also was discussed with staff through one-on-one conversations, in staff meetings, and at the unit practice council. Physicians attended the meetings as ad hoc members, and information was also shared through the operating room steering committee.

Selection

The team discussed and decided on pertinent issues, created a deployment list, and identified an action timeline for completion. Issues included the unexpected volume and case types that Surgical Services experienced, including the high volume in endoscopy and the inadequate environment for the recovery of the endoscopy patients. The deployment action items included the build-out of a new area for endoscopy patient recovery.

Testing

After implementing the changes and monitoring, the team began collecting data and measuring the effect of the interventions on the plan. The team was then able to act on the knowledge and select additional changes to implement or a replication plan, if indicated. The test was represented by the continuing review of Gallup scores that attained the goal set by the group. Further, the improvement in RN reports on the "Overall Had a Good Day" showed that the changes improved staff satisfaction as well (see Figure 3 on previous page).

The areas that improved BMCS Surgical Services staff satisfaction and "Overall Had a Good Day" included the following:

FIGURE 4.
FAST Performance Improvement Model

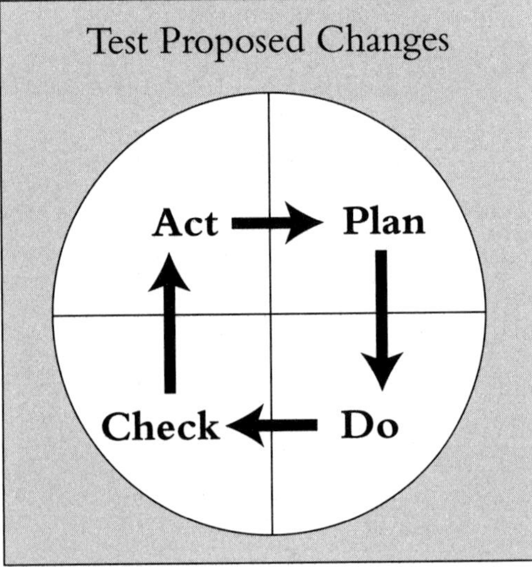

STEPS

Focus on a specific aim

- Specify an aim for the improvement project
- Set a numerical target for improvement

Analyze basic data

- Select and gather data for baseline measurement
- Compare baseline data with the target
- Determine key causes

Select potential changes

- Generate changes to test
- Decide on process changes or interventions to be made

Test the proposed changes

- Implement the changes and monitor
- Collect data and measure the effect of the interventions on the plan

Act on the knowledge gained

- Select additional changes to implement if indicated
- Develop an implementation and/or a replication plan
- Decide on need for further improvement or continue with monitoring plan
- Decide on actions to sustain the gain

- Developing a new assignment schedule that included specific staff assignments for pre- and post-endoscopy
- Installing an automatic door to the exit, to ease the process of staff moving patients in wheelchairs at time of discharge
- Establishing a process for call-outs so that appropriate staffing could be ensured
- Supplying additional computers for the unit and physician area
- Establishing a lunch and break relief process to support staff breaks and adequate rest periods
- Evaluating and ensuring safety in the parking area for staff coming in during off-hours

The BMCS Surgical Services department formed a performance improvement team to focus on staff satisfaction to increase patient satisfaction. Dissatisfiers were identified. The surgical services staff acknowledged the importance of meeting all BMCS customers' needs using evidence-based practice, safety, and satisfaction. Customers were identified as patients, caregivers, staff, physicians, and volunteers. A team made up of representatives from all surgical areas—the main operating room, Ambulatory Surgery Unit, Endoscopy, Post-Anesthesia Care Unit, Guest Services, finance, leadership, and performance improvement—met weekly to identify potential changes to practice.

Conclusions and Implications

BMCS encourages staff to participate in surveys, discussions, and activities and not let the dialogue end there. Members of nursing leadership take the feedback, truly listen to the needs of nursing staff, and implement changes. Nurses stay with BMCS because the organization's integrity flows down to each individual unit through shared leadership and a high level of communication.

The 3B MSP and Surgical Services units highlight the improvements made that affected the "Overall Had a Good Day" ratings in their respective areas. In addition, nurses were asked to identify what they believe makes a day good overall. A common theme emerged, with staff identifying nursing leadership, from the bedside to administration, as a key factor.

In both units, communication was key to the success of the implemented improvements. Staff are positive and supportive when they are involved and informed. Nursing leaders from the bedside to administration understand and care enough to know that listening is a key step in communication before action can be taken.

References

Baptist Health (July, 2008). The service excellence guide to the patient/family experience.

Benner, P. (1984) *From novice to expert: Excellence and power in clinical nursing practice.* Menlo Park: Addison-Wesley.

Redesigning Unit Orientation Improves Satisfaction for Nurses and Patients

Candice Herman, MSN, RN, NEA-BC
Director of Professional Development
candice.herman@mhbh.org

Beverly White, MBA/HCM, BSN, ADN, RNC
Administrative Director of Women's Services

Memorial Hermann Baptist Hospital—Beaumont, Texas

Editor's Pick

INSIGHTS & IDEAS FROM THIS FACILITY

Matching an orientee with a mentor who uses the orientee's learning style improves satisfaction with orientiation.

Facility and Unit Summary

Facility	Memorial Hermann Baptist Hospital (MHBH)—Beaumont, Texas **www.mhbh.org**
Facility setting	MHBH has served its communities for over 50 years, adding surgical, intensive care, pediatric, diagnostic, and outpatient services to the existing services, including rehabilitation and physical therapy, cancer services, comprehensive psychiatric services, and expanded expanded emergency department
Teaching status	Nonteaching hospital
Ownership status	Not-for-profit community hospital
Community demographics	Located 90 miles west of Houston, 30 miles east of Louisiana, and 30 miles north of the Gulf of Mexico, with a land area of 85 square miles; population 113,866 • White, non-Hispanic (46.4%) • Black (45.8%) • Hispanic (7.9%) • Other race (3.5%) • Approximately 13.6% of service area population age 65+
Hospital-staffed beds	330 beds
Case mix index	1.23
Indicators used	RN Satisfaction
System or unit improved	Labor and Delivery (L&D) and Post-Partum
Indicator improved	RN Satisfaction: Nurse Satisfaction with Unit Orientation
QI documents used	RN Satisfaction Survey
Time frame of QI experience	2005–2007
NDNQI® participation	Since 2005
Magnet™ status	Recognized September 2007
Governance model	Shared Governance

Awards and recognition	• Press Ganey Compass Award—2005, 2007 • Recognition For Disease-Specific Care: Stroke—2007 • Mimi Powell Huey Partnership Circle Award—2007 • Pathway to Excellence—2007 • Leadership Award for Excellence in Cardiac Care—2006 • Texas Health Care Quality Improvement Award—2005

UNIT PROFILE

L&D

Internal name	L&D (Labor & Delivery),
Size and type	7 labor beds; 4 triage beds; 2 operating rooms with 2-bed recovery; women's services unit
Staff summary	24 RNs; 7 certified scrub technicians (CSTs), 2 unit clerks (UCs); 1 birth registrar (BR)
Staff skill mix	70.6% RN; 20.6% CST; 5.9% UC; 2.9% BR
Nurse-patient ratio (NHPPD)	1:1, 1:2

PP

Internal name	PP (Post-Partum)
Size and type	Women's services unit: 27 beds
Staff summary	11 RNs; 7 licensed vocational nurses (LVNs); 1 unlicensed assistive personnel (UAP); 1 unit clerk; 1 childbirth educator
Staff skill mix	52.4% RN; 33.3% LVN; 4.8% UC; 4.8% UAP; 4.8% educator
Nurse-patient ratio (NHPPD)	1:6

Organizational structure	Director, Charge nurse, Staff

Redesigning Unit Orientation Improves Satisfaction for Nurses and Patients

Candice Herman, MSN, RN, NEA-BC
Beverly White, MBA/HCM, BSN, ADN, RNC

Memorial Hermann Baptist Hospital— Beaumont, Texas

Introductory Summary

Having an effective unit orientation and a strong preceptor program is essential to the recruitment and retention of staff nurses in today's market. In 2005, the new director for Women's Center services—which comprises two units, Labor and Delivery (L&D) and Post-Partum (PP)—quickly realized that, with a high RN vacancy rate and challenges to finding experienced perinatal nurses, improved recruitment and retention strategies had to be a priority.

Like many hospitals, Memorial Hermann Baptist Hospital (MHBH) had a unit orientation for new RNs and a formalized preceptor program for recent graduates. The nursing department, however, determined that these programs were not resulting in adequate support for RNs to transition from new hires to effective team members on all units. Communication and coping are necessary skills for any nurse, but they are essential to those caring for patients in the fast-paced and sometimes stressful environment of perinatal units. For perinatal nursing units to deliver safe quality patient care, the staff must be effective team members, in addition to being technically competent. The existing program did not incorporate the principal skills for being an effective team member. The orientation and preceptor programs were revised and strengthened not only to include a comprehensive orientation that prepared nurses to be competent in their roles; they prepared RNs also to be active members of a team by participating in shared governance and professional practice.

The new orientation program focused on four key concepts that must be integral for the new employee to successfully transition from being a *new hire* to being a member of the team with competent independent nursing practice. The four concepts are:

- Effective communication
- Tools to facilitate effective communication
- Positive role modeling
- Promotion of professional development and practice

One consequence of the revised orientation program was an increase in RN satisfaction with unit orientation. Creating a team environment through education, mentoring, and standardization of the evaluation process improved not only the satisfaction of nurses in the L&D and PP units (Figure 1), but also the satisfaction of the patients for whom they cared (Figure 2). Furthermore, the RN vacancy rate decreased dramatically on L&D.

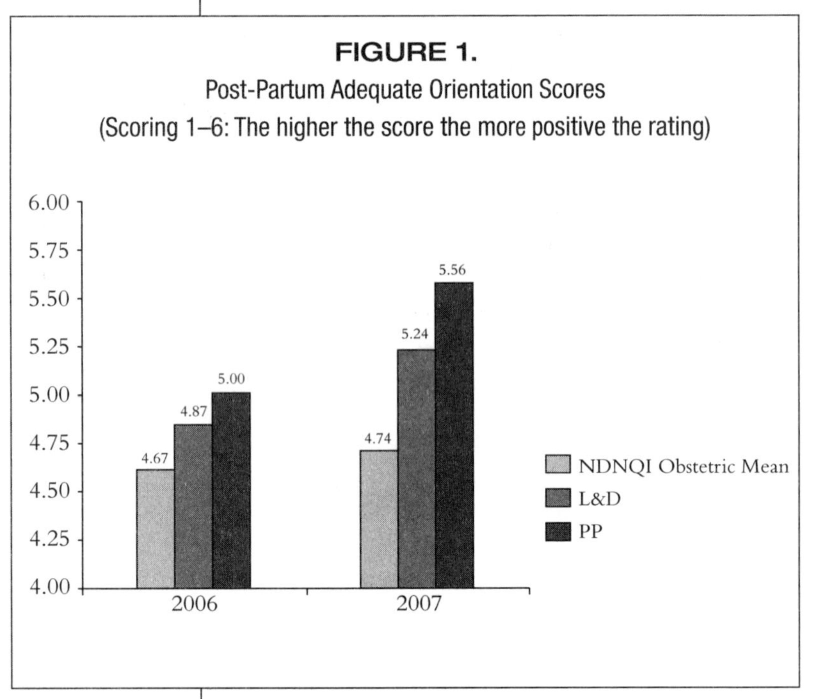

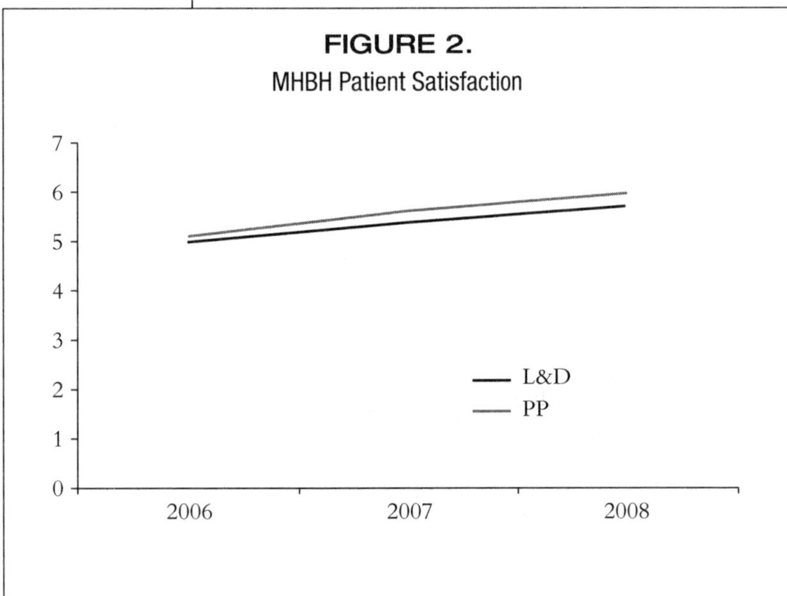

Background

In 2005, when MHBH first participated in the NDNQI RN Satisfaction Survey, the questionnaire did not specifically ask about the survey indicator measuring nurse satisfaction with unit orientation. However, it did give results on overall job enjoyment, with a wide range of scores across different units. Job enjoyment scores for L&D and Post-Partum were in the bottom 25% of the scores nationally. Because of the poor scores and high vacancy rate, nursing leadership explored contributing factors. Open discussions were held during staff meetings, and leaders interviewed individual staff members. Two common themes emerged: first, a work environment characterized by

- Poor communication among the team members, and
- No organized method to promote professional practice.

The existing competency-based orientation program was suitable for preparing new nurses with skills and knowledge needed to provide perinatal care; however, it was not adequately preparing them to be active members of a team. Preceptors were being selected based on tenure rather than on communication and teaching skills. Orientees were being placed with preceptors based on schedules rather than being matched on learning styles and personality. Compounding the orientation problem was the manner in which deficiencies were handled. It was common for physicians and staff alike to comment inappropriately on the performance of the orientee or the preceptor in public areas of nursing units, leading to decreased confidence and morale for both.

The competency-based orientation for L&D and Post-Partum was built on the Association of Women's Health, Obstetric and Neonatal Nurses (AWHONN) standards and provided a framework that combines knowledge and clinical skills verification. The orientation was divided into nine modules, with each module covering concepts, objectives, and a skills checklist that included topics such as organization of patient care, admission of the laboring patient, high-risk labor and delivery, and medication administration. The program encompassed a variety of teaching methods to meet the objectives of each module, including reading material, videotapes, classroom instruction, and clinical rotations through perioperative services and all of the Women's Services nursing units.

Additionally, the orientation program is tailored to the individual needs of the orientee, and the preceptor is given the autonomy to increase or decrease the pace based on the performance of the orientee. Some organizational elements changed to enhance the nurses' competency. Nurses are sent to a 2-day AWHONN fetal heart monitoring program during orientation when previously it was provided in-house by tenure nurses, and the Neonatal Resuscitation Program (NRP) is completed in the orientation period when previously it was required within 1 year of employment.

FIGURE 3.

Assessing Learning Styles: Suggested Interview Questions

1. In school did you prefer to get new information in:
   (a) Pictures, diagrams, graphs, or
   (b) Written directions, or
   (c) Verbal information
2. Do you believe that you remember best by:
   (a) What you see, or
   (b) What you hear
3. When learning a new skill, would you rather:
   (a) Try things out, or
   (b) Think about how it is done
4. Would you consider yourself:
   (a) Outgoing, or
   (b) More reserved

Redesign of the Orientation

The leadership team worked with the nursing staff to redesign the existing orientation program. First, the list of nurses who were preceptors was examined closely. Several nurses had been chosen to be preceptors based on their tenure on the unit rather than on their ability to teach. After these nurses' interactions with co-workers were observed and staff input was solicited, some preceptors were removed from the role and new preceptors were recruited. Staff members were identified who demonstrated the clinical skills and teaching skills necessary to be effective preceptors. Specific communication tools and processes were developed to enhance the orientation experience between the preceptor, new employee, and director.

The learning styles of job candidates are assessed during the interview process. In addition to the standard behavioral interview questions, the interview team asks a few questions specifically related to learning preferences. Staff participating in the interview and selection process also identify the most appropriate preceptor for new employees. The selection is based on trying to match the preferred learning style of the new employee with the teaching style of the preceptor. (See Figure 3 for the interview questions.)

Experienced preceptors provided feedback to the team designing and implementing the new orientation program and identified that the most positive change to the orientation process was how feedback was handled. A formal evaluation process was created to allow the preceptor and the orientee the opportunity to evaluate each other in a safe, comfortable environment. Now employees evaluate their experiences independently and then submit their evaluations to the director, who reviews them prior to meeting with employees (Figure 4).

To ensure that both the orientee and the preceptor are being successful, the director meets with them first individually and then together to discuss the orientation experiences, accomplishments, challenges, and goals for the new hire. These meetings enhance communication, provide encouragement, give constructive feedback, and celebrate accomplishments. During the joint meeting, the director discusses the positives, and if any deficiencies are identified, they are discussed in a nonthreatening manner. Initially the meetings are weekly for approximately 4 to 6 weeks, then biweekly for 3 to 6 weeks, and then they conclude with a final meeting at the end of the 3-month orientation period. Occasionally, the frequency of the meetings may vary depending on the orientation progress of the new hire.

FIGURE 4.

Orientee's Evaluation of Preceptor

Date: ______________________

Name: ______________________

Preceptor: ______________________

Goals set for the week by preceptor:

1. ______________________
2. ______________________
3. ______________________

Goals accomplished:

1. ______________________
2. ______________________
3. ______________________

What was the most positive experience this week? ______________________

____

What was the least positive experience this week? ______________________

____

Goals for the upcoming week(s)

1. ______________________
2. ______________________
3. ______________________

Please rate your preceptor based on the following criteria: 5= Excellent, 4= Good, 3= Satisfactory, 2= Needs improvement, 1= Unsatisfactory, NA= Unable to evaluate (requires explanation)

	5	4	3	2	1	N/A
Was readily available to you						
Assigned tasks/skills consistent with your level of experience/training						
Provided clear direction/expectation about assigned skills						
Provided constructive feedback regarding your performance						
Expressed positive attitude						
Encouraged questions						
Communicated clinical knowledge well						
Provided alternative experience when presented						
Encouraged your participation						

As noted above, the confidence of orientees and preceptors was being undermined by physician and staff comments in public spaces. To address this issue, the director met individually with physicians to discuss the changes and goal of moving the culture and environment to one that embraces learning through a positive and welcoming atmosphere. Subsequent to the meeting, any concerns about the nurse's performance or progress were given directly to the director to address, and not to the new employee or the preceptor. This change in process has resulted in more professional interactions between physicians and nurses. Physicians and nurses treat each other with more respect, with less blaming, and the communication remains focused on patient care, all reinforcing the team environment.

FIGURE 5.

Post-Partum, RN Turnover Rates (percent)

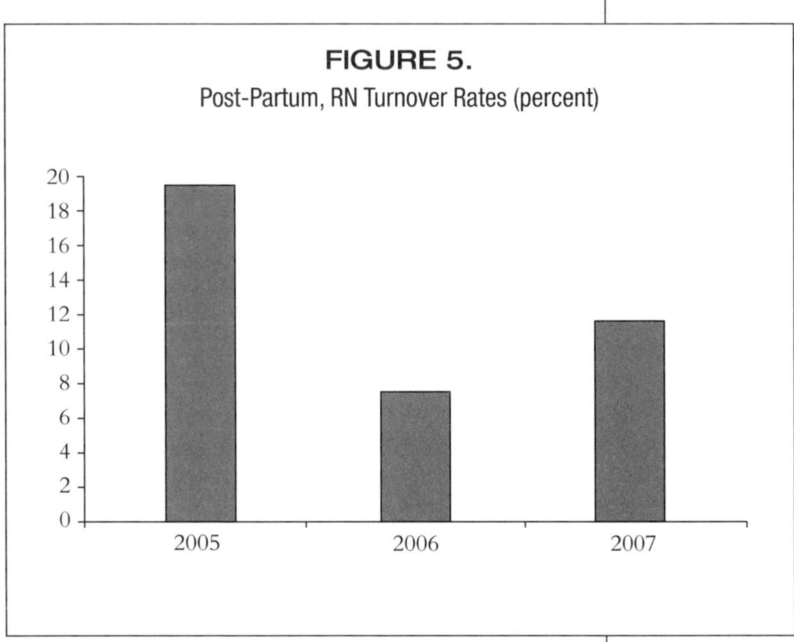

Consequences

The primary goal for the revised orientation program was to decrease vacancy rates and prepare inexperienced nurses to provide quality patient care to the ob/gyn population. In the first year after the revisions, the RN vacancy rate decreased from 10.82% on L&D to 2.94% and has been at 0% since June 2006. Each semester there is a list of new graduate nurses who desire to gain a position in Post-Partum. Although turnover on this unit has not been eliminated completely, the turnover rate decreased from 19.52% in 2005 to 11.85% in 2007 (Figure 5). While an increase in nurse satisfaction with the redesigned program was anticipated, the speed and degree of improvement exceeded expectations.

An unexpected result of the revised program has been an increase in the sense of pride among the staff nurses and their desire to project a more professional nursing image. The unit-based shared governance council approached the director in September 2006 with an idea to start a local AWHONN chapter. By 2008, there were 12 nurses from MHBH that were active members of the new Southeast Texas Beaumont Chapter, and 7 of 8 elected officers were MHBH employees. Preceptors encourage orientees to become involved in the chapter and invite them to attend at least one chapter meeting during the orientation period. The feedback from the preceptors and the orientees has been that encouraging professional development in orientation results in social networking and facilitates inclusion in the team. The local AWHONN chapter started a pay-it-forward program to assist new nurses by paying the fee for national certification. The chapter will pay the initial fee on behalf of the new staff member. Once the employee receives reimbursement, he or she then repays the chapter's certification fund.

A significant relationship has been found between nurses' positive perception of their work environment and higher patient satisfaction (Donahue, Piazza, Griffin, Dykes, & Fitzpatrick, 2008). The MHBH experience with the revised nursing orientation program (the form in Figure 6 is part of this) also resulted in an increase in the patient satisfaction scores in Women's Services, demonstrating that an engaged workforce results in better patient satisfaction (as shown in Figure 2).

FIGURE 6.
Case Scenarios

The charge nurse notifies you that you are going to be admitting the new patient that is arriving. Wanting to be organized and prepared you find the:

❑ Prenatal record ❑ Baby bracelets ❑ Admission chart packet

You proceed to the labor room to check that it is stocked with all needed supplies. You observe that you are missing a few things. Please find:

❑ O2 mask ❑ Boston hat ❑ Monitor belts ❑ Pt belongings bag ❑ KY jelly ❑ Nonsterile gloves

You also notice that your chart is not complete. Please find:

❑ Glossy Slick sheet ❑ Consent forms

When the patient arrives, it is obvious that she will need to be admitted promptly. Please find:

❑ Enema set ❑ IV solutions ❑ IV tubing ❑ IV start kits/tray

After the patient returns to bed from expelling her enema she states that she thinks her "water broke." You see no obvious fluid, so you will need to check:

❑ Sterile speculum ❑ Glass slide ❑ Sterile swap ❑ Slide jacket

The patient is now very uncomfortable and she is requesting an epidural. Please find:

❑ Anesthesia cart ❑ Pyxis ❑ Epidural infusion pump ❑ EKG monitor ❑ NIBP monitor ❑ Anesthesia supply cabinet ❑ Tape ❑ Anesthesia record

Your patient is now delivering and the doctor is asking for all kinds of things. Please find:

❑ Simpson forceps ❑ Vacuum ❑ Curette ❑ Biogel sterile gloves ❑ Stool ❑ Shoe covers ❑ Hemabate ❑ Mask

You notice that the baby is blue. Please find:

❑ Emergency call bell ❑ Laryngoscope with blade ❑ Ambo bag ❑ Delee suction ❑ Bulb syringe ❑ Warm blankets

Your patient had a c-section and is now in the recovery phase, and the anesthesiologist begins to request items. Please find:

❑ Nebulizer bottle ❑ ET tube ❑ Suction tubing ❑ Face shield ❑ Corrugated tubing ❑ Blood tubing ❑ Oral airway ❑ EKG pads ❑ Fluid warmer ❑ Yankaur suction ❑ Normal saline ❑ Bear hugger

CONGRATULATIONS! You transferred your patient to Post-Partum. Please find:

❑ Break room ❑ Coffee ❑ A place to sit ❑ Snack

Conclusion and Implications

Diffusion of innovation theory provided a useful perspective for MHBH about the challenges to be faced in adopting new processes associated with the redesigned orientation. According to Rogers (2003), those changes that are perceived as having the greatest relative advantage will be adopted more rapidly. As might be expected, the orientation program changes generated some resistance among a few of the more experienced nurses, especially those who had been removed as preceptors. Overall, the changes were well received by nursing staff and, based on the positive outcomes, were well worth the effort.

In the future, the orientation programs for all nursing areas will incorporate the communication tools used by the Women's Services departments. As nurses continue to see the value of effective communication between the orientees, preceptors, managers, and physicians, and how communication can positively influence their own satisfaction in the workplace, additional advances in nurse recruitment and retention can be envisioned.

References

Donahue, M. O., Piazza, I. M., Griffin, M. Q., Dykes, P. C., & Fitzpatrick, J. J. (2008). The relationship between nurses' perceptions of empowerment and patient satisfaction. *Applied Nursing Research, 21*, 2–7. doi: 10.1016/j.apnr.2007.11.001.

Rogers, E. (2003). *Diffusion of innovations* (5th ed.). New York: Free Press.

Making the Connection between RN Satisfaction and RN Retention

Marianne J. Harkin, BSN, MS, RN, CNRN
Project Director of Nursing Quality
Marianne.Harkin@nyumc.org

Pam Brown, RN, MA
Director of Nursing, Compliance and Risk Management

Joan M. Cutrone, MA, RN, CPN, LNC, NEA-BC
Nurse Manager, Neonatal Intensive Care Unit

Bernadette Daborn, RN, MA, CPNP
Nurse Manager, Pediatric Intensive Care Unit

Jeanne Dzurenko, RN, MPH
Director of Nursing, Rusk Institute of Rehabilitation Medicine, Psychiatry, and Radiology

Susan Frost, CRNA, BS
Chief CRNA

Karen Goodman, MA, RN, IBCLC, LCCE
Nurse Manager, Mother–Baby Unit

Marge Lilienthal, RN, MS, NEA-BC
Director of Nursing, Maternal Child Services

Arlene McGee, RN, MA/MS
Nurse Manager, Cardiopulmonary Rehabilitation Unit

Megan Tateishi, CRNA, MS
Assistant Chief CRNA

New York University Hospitals Center

Editor's Pick

INSIGHTS & IDEAS FROM THIS FACILITY

While nurse managers foster teamwork, they in turn are supported through a Nurse Manager Wellness Program, which includes an emphasis on "mindfulness" being in the moment.

Facility and Unit Summary

Facility	NYU Hospitals Center—New York, NY **www.med.nyu.edu**
Facility setting	Full complement of services with areas of specialization in cardiovascular services, oncology, neuroscience, musculoskeletal, rehabilitation, and ambulatory surgery.
Teaching status	Academic medical center
Ownership status	Nonprofit
Community demographics	• Serves a diverse cultural population of patients within the tristate area (several boroughs and counties of New York, New Jersey, and Connecticut) • Approx. 11.5% of service area population over age 65.
Hospital-staffed beds	655 staffed beds
Case mix index (CMI)	1.81
Indicators used	RN Survey: Job Plans
System or units improved	RN Satisfaction: High percentage of staff wanting to stay on their same unit in the same position. The units: • PICU (Pediatric Intensive Care Unit) • NICU (Neonatal Intensive Care Unit) • 13 West (Mother–Baby) • HCC 9 (Cardiopulmonary Rehabilitation) • OR CRNA (Certified Registered Nurse Anesthetists)
Indicator improved	Unit RN job plans for the next year: Stay in my current position
QI documents used	RN Survey Reports
NDNQI® participation	Since Q3-02
Time frame of QI experience	2005–2007
Magnet™ status	Since March 2005
Governance model	Participatory Leadership Structure
Awards and recognition	• U.S. News and World Report Best Hospitals Honor Roll • Leapfrog Top 26 Hospitals 2008

UNIT PROFILES

PICU

Internal name	PICU (Pediatric Intensive Care Unit)
Size and type	13-bed critical care unit caring for pediatric patients from infancy to 18 years of age; predominately a surgical critical care unit caring for neurosurgical, cardiac, orthopedic, urology, epilepsy, and general pediatric surgical patients as well as some medical patients
Staff summary	Staffed by all RNs (23), with a support staff of 2 evening/night assistant nurse managers, patient unit clerks, and a supply aid
Staff skill mix	• All RNs; certifications 11% • Education: DIPN, 6.7 %; BSN, 77.3 %; MSN, 20%
Nurse-patient ratio (NHPPD)	14 NHPPD (1:1–1:3)
Organizational structure	Nurse manager, assistant nurse managers, nursing staff (RNs, supply aid); the nurse manager has 24-hour, 7-day-a-week responsibility for a unit's nursing care; unit-based assistant nurse managers on evenings and nights support the unit nursing staff

NICU

Internal name	NICU (Neonatal Intensive Care Unit)
Size and type	25-bed Level III unit with 3 designated neonatal intensive care beds
Staff summary	Staffed by all RNs (42, including the nurse manager and 2 evening/night assistant nurse managers), with a support staff of 1 supply aid
Staff skill mix	• All RNs; certifications 27% • Education: AAN, 4.1%; DIPN, 2.0%; BSN, 81.6%; MSN, 12.2%
Nurse-patient ratio (NHPPD)	9.67 average
Organizational structure	Nurse manager, Assistant nurse managers, Nursing staff

13 WEST

Internal name	13 West (Mother–Baby Unit)
Size and type	36 beds; family-centered mother–baby care; includes both a Level 1 Newborn Nursery, consisting of a transitional nursery for infants newly admitted to the Mother–Baby Unit from Labor and Delivery, and a Respite Nursery
Staff summary	• 54.2 RNs • 3 LPNs • 16.5 Nursing attendants
Staff skill mix	• Certification of RNs, 21% • Education: AAN, 1.6%; DIPN, 3.2%; BSN, 90.5%; MSN, 4.8%
Nurse–patient ratio (NHPPD)	6.8 average NHPPD to the mother and baby
Organizational structure	Nurse manager, Assistant nurse managers, Nursing staff

HCC 9

Internal name	HCC 9 (Cardiopulmonary Rehabilitation)
Size and type	22-bed unit; provides rehabilitation to postoperative cardiac and pulmonary surgical patients and selected cardiac and pulmonary medical patients
Staff summary	• 15 RNs • 10 nursing attendants • TBD LPNs (who float within the rehabilitation service)
Staff skill mix	Certifications: • RNs: TBD • LPNs: TBD Education: • RNs: TBD • LPNs: TBD
Nurse–patient ratio (NHPPD)	• RNs: 5.9 • Nursing attendants: 2.6 • LPNs: 0.04
Organizational structure	Nurse manager, Clinical coordinator, Nursing staff

OR CRNA

Internal name	OR CRNA (Operating Room Certified Registered Nurse Anesthetists)
Size and type	Acute care hospital with 51 operative suites providing approximately 3,000 procedures per month; anesthesiology, the administration of anesthesia, and the education of student nurse anesthetists
Staff summary	19 CRNAs
Staff skill mix	Per certification and education requirements for CRNAs
Nurse-patient ratio (NHPPD)	Not applicable
Organizational structure	Chief of Service (Anesthesia Department), Chief CRNA, Staff CRNAs

Making the Connection between RN Satisfaction and RN Retention

Marianne J. Harkin, BSN, MS, RN, CNRN
Pam Brown, RN, MA
Joan M. Cutrone, MA, RN, CPN, LNC, NEA-BC
Bernadette Daborn, RN, MA, CPNP
Jeanne Dzurenko, RN, MPH
Susan Frost, CRNA, BS
Karen Goodman, MA, RN, IBCLC, LCCE
Marge Lilienthal, RN, MS, NEA-BC
Arlene McGee, RN, MA/MS
Megan Tateishi, CRNA, MS

New York University Hospitals Center

Introductory Summary

NYU Hospitals Center (NYUHC) is an academic medical center in New York City that includes Tisch Hospital for acute care and Rusk Institute of Rehabilitation Medicine, an acute inpatient rehabilitation hospital. Participation in the National Database of Nursing Indicators (NDNQI) RN Satisfaction Survey began in 2003, and Magnet™ designation was attained in March 2005.

NYUHC offers the NDNQI RN Satisfaction Survey to RNs to identify issues affecting job satisfaction. August 2008 marked the sixth year that NYUHC has administered this survey. At NYUHC, the survey response rate has increased over time. In 2007, the response rate was 82%, notably higher than the 75% rate in 2006. The favorable increase in response was due to the perceived value of the survey and its role in influencing improvement initiatives based on findings.

The demographics of the RN respondents at NYUHC differ from the overall NDNQI survey respondents in two major categories. The educational achievements NYUHC RNs were well above the NDNQI peer group comparison in terms of educational attainment (Table 1).

The second major difference was related to the average age. Across NYUHC units, on average, 29% of respondents were below age 30 compared with 18% for the NDNQI benchmark; 39% were over the age of 40 compared with 57% for NDNQI. Overall, the average age of RNs on NYUHC units who responded to the survey was 39 years, compared with 43 years for all NDNQI.

At NYUHC, the RN Satisfaction Survey has been an invaluable tool. Unit-level results were analyzed to determine unit-specific action plans to improve and/or sustain RN retention. The analysis of the sur-

TABLE 1.
RN Education at NYUHC

	Nursing Degree (%)		Non-Nursing Degree (%)	
Degree	NDNQI	NYUHC	NDNQI	NYUHC
Diploma	12	5	——	——
AD	38	5	16	5
BSN	46	71	20	30
MS/PhD	4	19	3	6

vey findings has become more sophisticated over the past 4 years. For the 2006 and 2007 survey results, a data analyst consultant was used to "drill down" into the data and identify trends. An in-depth summary of findings was prepared, which included comparative data from previous years, and reviewed with the Executive Nursing Council. The results were depicted at the service and unit levels in a format that was easy to digest and allowed the reader to quickly identify trends and variances. The format included a dashboard (Table 2) by service as well as graphs that highlighted significant findings. These reports were shared with unit-level leadership and RN staff and were used as a springboard for the development of initiatives to improve RN satisfaction at the unit level. An example of the type and format of information provided by the consultant is depicted in Table 2.

The value of the survey supported the adage applicable to many hospital systems: "You can only manage what you can measure." Knowing about high, moderate, or low satisfaction among RNs at NYUHC was essential for nursing management and staff to design strategies for improving job satisfaction and retaining staff. The nurses understood this process and demonstrated, by their survey response, enthusiastic support of the goals that NDNQI represented.

One of the positive findings identified was that five patient care units had a high percentage of RNs who intended to remain working on their home units, a result that has been sustained for at least the past 3 years (Figure 1). The units are diverse, but the work satisfaction issues are extremely similar. The units include Pediatric Intensive Care (PICU), Neonatal Intensive Care (NICU), Mother–Baby Unit, Cardiopulmonary Rehabilitation, and the Certified Registered Nurse Anesthetists (CRNA) group.

Of all the reasons for high retention on these units, the predominant theme was that the units had enculturated a sense of family among the staff. The leadership style fostered autonomy of nursing practice, self-scheduling, work–life balance, teamwork, and collaboration. In comparison with the younger average age of the nursing staff, the tenure of the nurse managers of the five identified units was long. Unit management tenure ranged from 8 to 30 years.

One of the factors that contributed to the ability of the nurse managers to foster teamwork on their respective units was the initiation of the Nurse Manager Wellness Program by the Nursing Education Department. The program, which exemplifies quality of nursing leadership and management style (two of the 14 "Forces of Magnetism"), promoted nursing excellence on a personal and organizational level. The program goal was to reduce stress and promote leadership effectiveness through the practice of mindfulness. This practice of moment-to-moment awareness resulted in a profound shift in managers' understanding of themselves and others, allowing for an increase in respectful and trusting communication.

The nurse managers of the Mother–Baby Unit, the NICU, the PICU, and the Cardiopulmonary Reha-

TABLE 2.

Interpretation of Work Satisfaction *T*-Scores: NDNQI and Nursing Units, Maternal Child Service 2007

Work Satisfaction Measures	NDNQI: Obstetrics	13 West	8 E/W	NDNQI: Neonate	NICU	NDNQI: Pediatrics	9 East	PICU	Hassenfeld
Aggregate Unit Measures									
Task	Moderate	Low	Low	Moderate	Moderate	Moderate	Moderate	High	Moderate
RN–RN Interactions	High	High	High	High	High	High	High	High	High
RN–MD Interactions	Moderate	Moderate	Moderate	High	High	High	Moderate	High	Moderate
Decision-Making	Moderate	Moderate	Moderate	Moderate	Moderate	Moderate	Moderate	Moderate	Moderate
Automony	Moderate	Moderate	Moderate	Moderate	Moderate	Moderate	Moderate	High	Moderate
Professional Status	High	Moderate	Moderate	High	High	High	High	High	High
Pay	Moderate	Low	Moderate	Moderate	Low	Moderate	Moderate	Moderate	Moderate
Job Enjoyment	Moderate	Moderate	Low	Moderate	High	Moderate	Moderate	High	Moderate
Professional Development	High	High	Moderate	High	High	High	High	High	Moderate
Nursing Management	Moderate	Moderate	Moderate	Moderate	High	Moderate	Moderate	High	High
Nursing Administration	Moderate	Moderate	Moderate	Moderate	Moderate	Moderate	Moderate	Moderate	High
Individual-Focused Measures									
Time for patient care	Moderate	Low	Moderate	Moderate	High	Moderate	Moderate	High	Moderate
Teamwork between coworkers	High	High	High	High	High	High	High	High	High
Physicians appeciate what I do	High	Moderate	Moderate	High	High	High	Moderate	High	High
Participate in decision-making	Moderate	Moderate	Moderate	Moderate	Moderate	Moderate	Moderate	Moderate	Moderate
Autonomy in daily practice	Moderate	Moderate	Moderate	Moderate	Moderate	Moderate	Moderate	Moderate	Moderate
Satisfied with status of nursing	Moderate	Moderate	Moderate	Moderate	High	Moderate	Moderate	High	High
Salary is satisfactory	Moderate	Moderate	Moderate	Moderate	Moderate	Moderate	Moderate	Moderate	Moderate
Satisfied with my job	High	Moderate	Moderate	High	High	High	High	High	High
Career development opportunities	High	High	Moderate	High	High	High	High	High	Moderate
Nurse manager is a good leader	Moderate	Moderate	Moderate	Moderate	High	High	Moderate	High	High
Satisfied with CNO	Moderate	Moderate	Moderate	Moderate	Moderate	Moderate	Moderate	Moderate	High
Total # High Scores	7	4	2	8	13	9	6	15	10
Total # Moderate Scores	15	15	18	14	8	13	16	7	12
Total # Low Scores	0	3	2	0	1	0	0	0	0

bilitation Unit participated in this voluntary program at NYUHC. Outcomes identified by participants included enhancements in the following areas: ability to focus, sense of control, and job enjoyment. They also experienced a less judgmental approach when dealing with staff issues and enhanced their listening skills. This led to a circle of trust, which supported a healthful work and practice environment. One of the nurse manager participants stated, "I am less judgmental and have increased tolerance. I am more mindful in my communications. I now encourage the staff to stop, think, and take a breath."

Comments from staff on these four units included: "I like the fairness of my Nurse Manager; she is always flexible with all the staff on the unit, and she is a strong leader"; and "The Nurse Manager is sensitive to work/life balance."

FIGURE 1

Percent of RNs Who Plan To Remain On Same Unit, 2005–2007

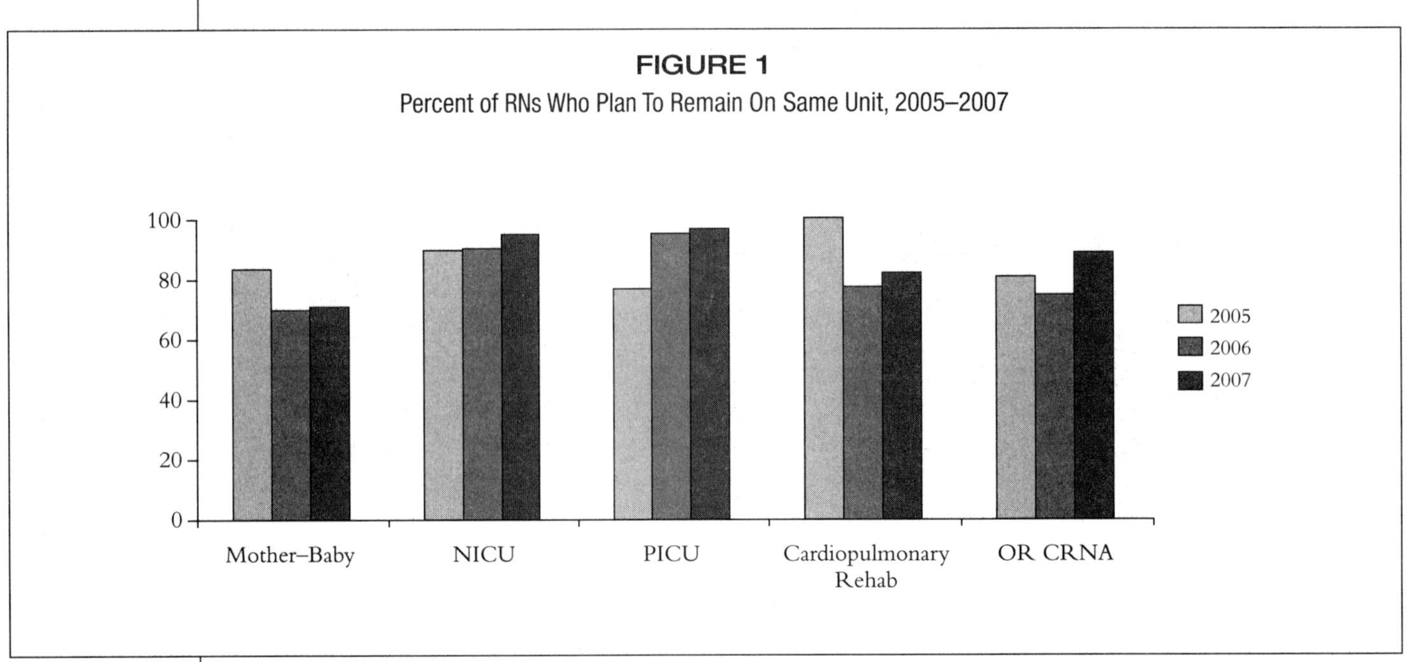

FIGURE 2

Percent of RNs Who Agree that Nurse Manager Is a Good Leader

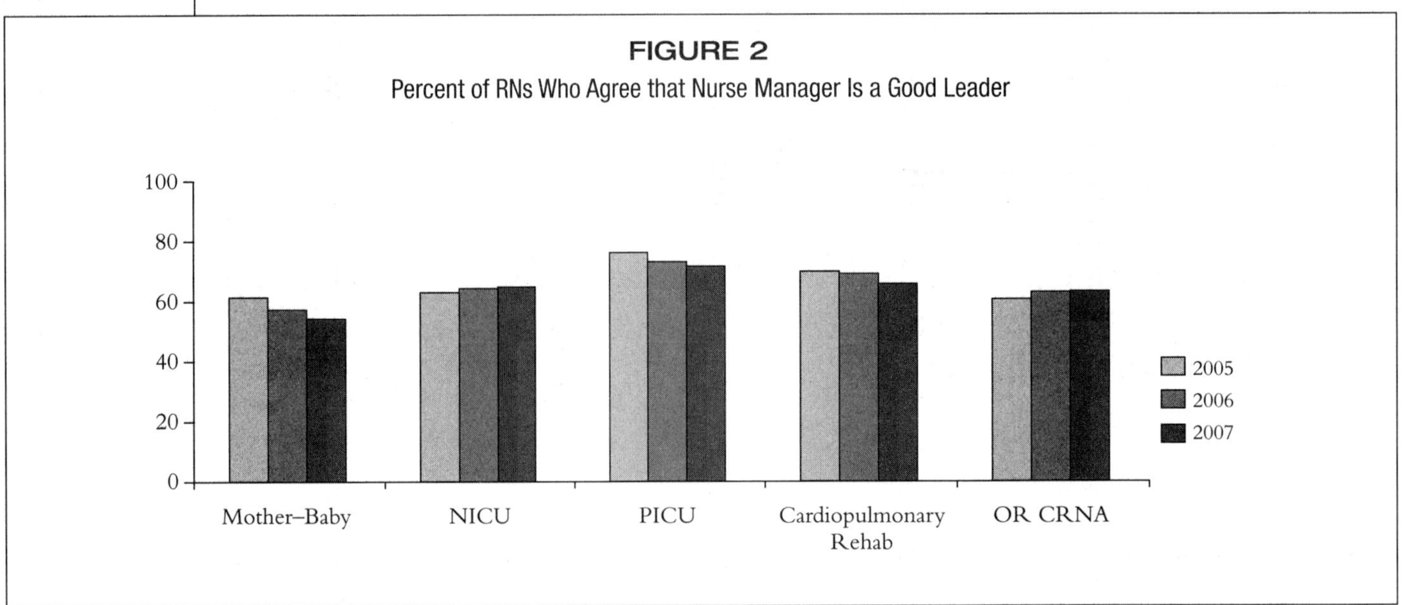

The concept of family, identified by the staff of these units as central to their desire to remain working on these units, can be exemplified by the following actual scenarios. The NICU staff describe the "swarm," where other RN staff come over to assist the RN who is admitting a neonate to the unit. This is a routine practice in the NICU so that no one RN feels she has to admit a new neonate alone. It exemplifies the concept of "many hands make light work." One of the NICU RNs stated: "I feel we are strong in team spirit, we work well together, pick up the ball for each other, and this helps make the day a whole lot easier."

The CRNA group also reported that teamwork was a very strong job satisfier for them, even though their work environment is very different from a typical patient care unit. Each certified registered nurse anesthetist is assigned individually to an operating room and doesn't work in the same room with other CRNAs. Their sense of teamwork is on a different level—both

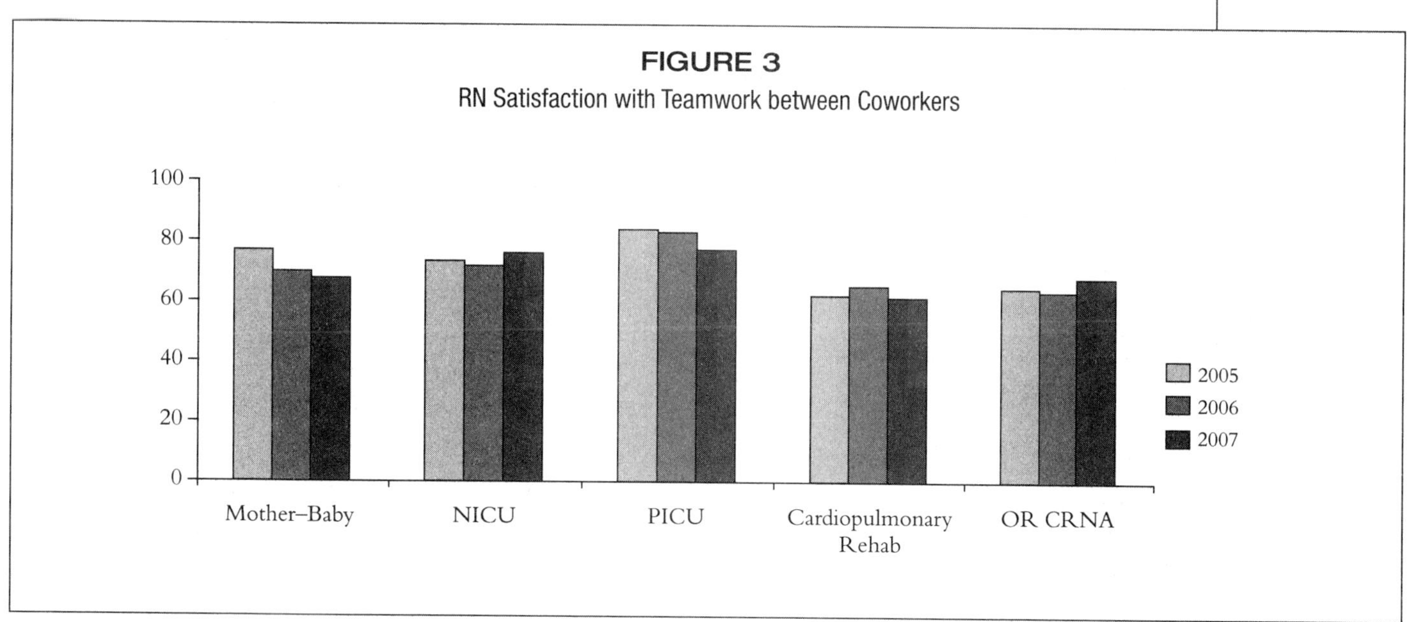

FIGURE 3
RN Satisfaction with Teamwork between Coworkers

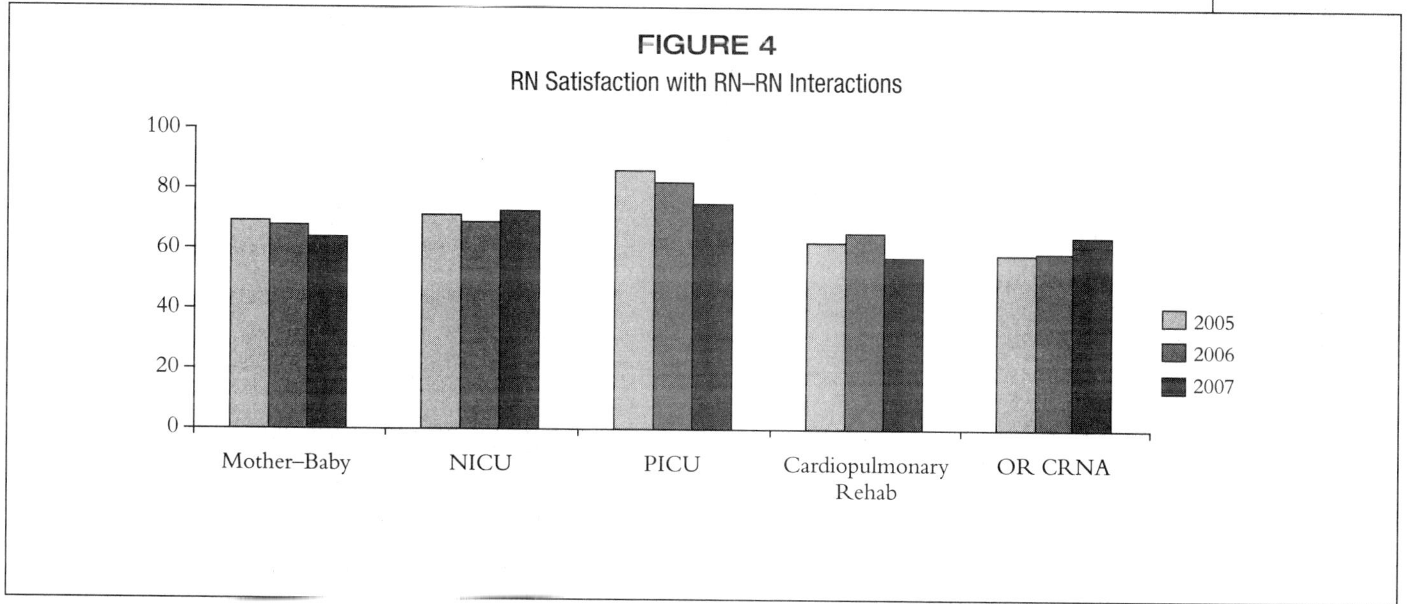

FIGURE 4
RN Satisfaction with RN–RN Interactions

professional and personal. Members of this group serve on the board of directors or as officers of national, state, or local professional associations. Coworkers show support by volunteering for various committees within these organizations to enlist speakers, sponsors, caterers, or help with registration at educational meetings. During a weekend state meeting, an NYUHC CRNA, who was committee chair, was rushed to the hospital. One of her NYUHC colleagues assumed her duties at the meeting and went to her home to take care of her cat. While they have minimal contact at work, the group functions as a team, covering shifts so others can attend educational meetings or travel to see family. They frequently socialize outside of work and consider each other a true support network. The strong feelings of teamwork between coworkers and the collegiality of the RN staff was validated through the responses to the related questions in the NDNQI survey as demonstrated in Figures 3 and 4.

The PICU staff described their feeling of family as interdisciplinary, with this example of teamwork

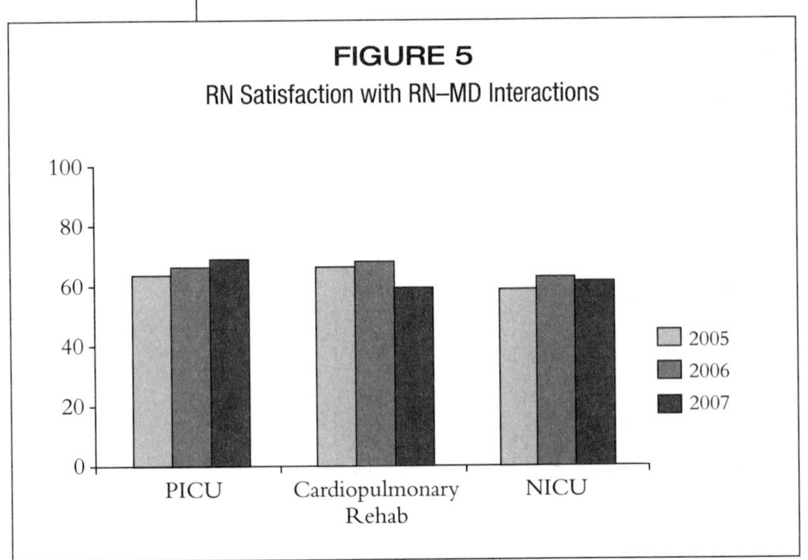

FIGURE 5
RN Satisfaction with RN–MD Interactions

between the MD and RN staff: as the PICU intensivist was leaving the building after a meeting, a pediatrician ran into her and told her, "They could use your help, a sick-looking infant was just brought into the Emergency Department." The intensivist went to the ED to help, the PICU was called for additional assistance, and two PICU nurses went to the ED. The team stabilized the baby and transferred her to the PICU. The infant was diagnosed with a life-threatening cardiac abnormality that required surgical repair. The baby experienced a successful, positive outcome and was discharged home, healthy and content, along with her parents.

The Cardiopulmonary Rehabilitation Unit is also proud of the extremely strong working relationship between the RNs and MDs and the obvious respect shown by the medical staff for the clinical knowledge of the RN staff. The attending physicians made it a point to tell each new group of residents that they must respond immediately when the RNs on the unit call with a change in a patient's condition. The clinical expertise of the RN staff is beyond measure. This message is reinforced during daily rounds, and the attending will counsel any resident who is not respectful to the RN staff. Additionally, the attending physicians have publicly acknowledged RN contributions as patient advocates and thanked them for their individual efforts in providing quality patient care. The positive RN–MD relationships on these units was consistent with the response to the related question in the RN Satisfaction Survey, as demonstrated in Figure 5.

Focused efforts by hospital administration were implemented to improve RN–MD communication and to foster mutual respect; thus, it was gratifying to see that there has been a measurable increase in RN satisfaction around this important measure.

One of the major factors affecting the desire of staff RNs to continue working on the Mother–Baby Unit was the identification by hospital and nursing leadership of the need to enhance the professional model of care delivery. It was recognized that there was a need to modify staffing patterns based upon guidelines of the American College of Obstetricians and Gynecologists, American Academy of Pediatrics, and Association of Women's Health Obstetric and Neonatal Nurses (AWHONN) guidelines. This model of care is designed to enhance the RN-to-patient ratio to provide 1 RN to 3.5 mother–baby couplets (1:3.5) in addition to the RN assigned as charge nurse. A 2-year implementation period resulted in additional registered nurse positions and a decrease in nursing attendant positions. There also was a strong emphasis on orientation of the new RN staff and relocation of the displaced nursing attendants to other units.

Finally, a critical factor that influenced the desire of staff to remain on a unit was the quality of the orientation experience. As noted earlier, NYUHC has a younger workforce, and a large percentage of the annual new hires are graduate nurses. The NYUHC Nurse Residency Program was established in 1996 and was designed to assist new BSN graduates as they transition into their first professional role in an acute care setting. It is a 1-year program in which all newly hired BSN graduates at NYUHC must participate. The program includes a series of learning and work experiences that provide the necessary tools for a smooth transition from the role of a student to the professional role. The graduate nurse is assigned to work on a specific unit for the entire year and is encouraged to

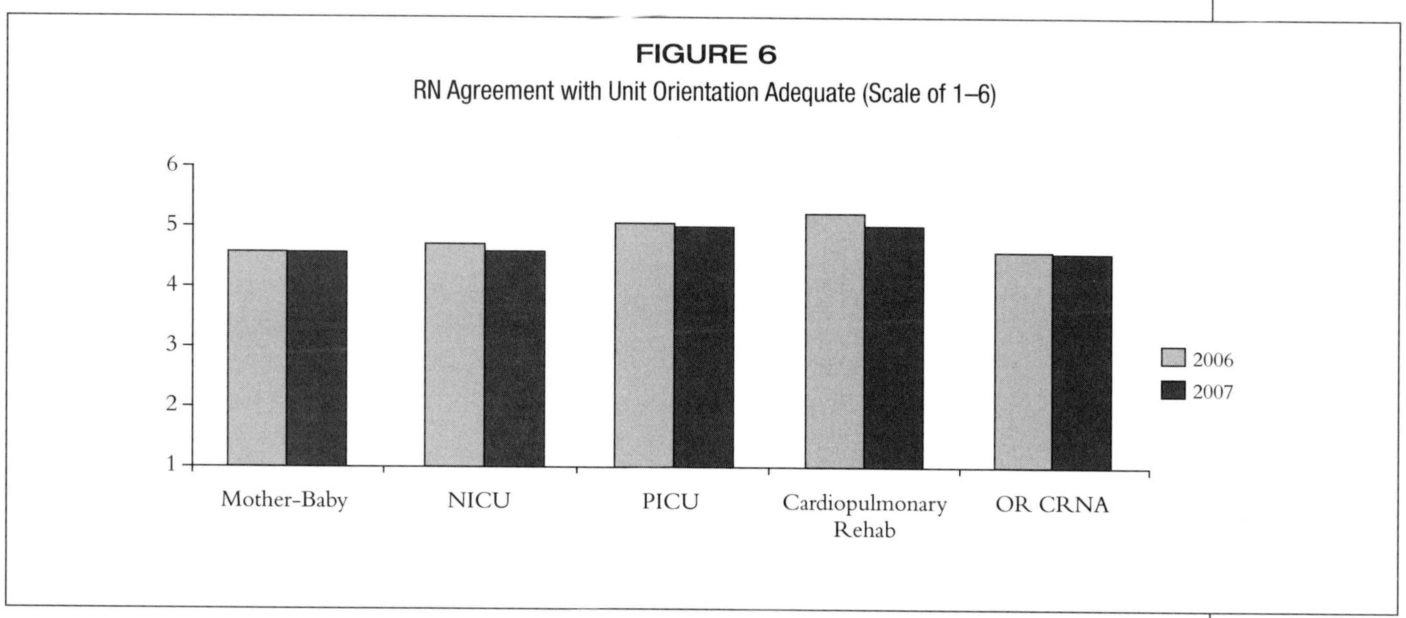

FIGURE 6

RN Agreement with Unit Orientation Adequate (Scale of 1–6)

remain a member of that nursing staff after the first year. Challenging clinical practice in an environment committed to learning is the key component of the Nurse Residency Program. Critical to the successful transition is the support the new graduate receives from senior staff and the nursing leadership of her or his unit. The new graduate functions as a full-time staff nurse, assuming all responsibilities appropriate for a first-year clinician, and actively participates in learning experiences with a consistent group of new BSN hires. Staff perceptions regarding adequacy of orientation are reflected in responses to the related question in the NDNQI survey (Figure 6.)

The review of the NDNQI RN Satisfaction Survey provided NYUHC with invaluable information regarding factors that positively influence RN retention, specifically the RNs' desire to continue to work on a particular unit. The analysis of the data from the survey over the past 3 years highlighted the importance of three key indicators that correlate strongly with job satisfaction. These include the influence of positive leadership at the unit level ("My nurse manager is a good leader"), the strength of positive interpersonal relationships (teamwork between coworkers, RN–RN interactions, and RN–MD interactions), and the investment of time in a meaningful orientation program ("Orientation is adequate"). The data demonstrated that taking the time to develop a unit culture that values and fosters teamwork, management support, and positive interpersonal relationships (both at the professional and personal level) has yielded a reward that is priceless—high retention at the unit level.

The positive results of the high retention level include the ability of nursing leadership and the unit to focus on quality and patient care initiatives rather than on continual recruitment and orientation of new staff. An additional benefit from improved retention was financial; recent estimates calculate the cost of replacing and retraining an RN at between 75% and 125% of the RN's annual salary, as reported by Beecroft, Kunzman, and Krozek (2001). This includes costs related to recruitment, overtime compensation to ensure coverage, orientation of replacement employees, lost productivity, and customer satisfaction.

NYUHC's goal is to be able to use the survey findings and knowledge gained from analysis to replicate this culture on other units. Plans are under way to explore the relationship between unit-level retention and unit-level patient outcomes (patient satisfaction and select nurse-sensitive indicators).

References

Beecroft P, Kunzman, L., & Krozek, C. (2001). RN internship: Outcomes of a one-year pilot program. *Journal of Nursing Administration, 31*(12), 575–582.

Additional Resources

Burns, S. M., & Hutchens, A. L. (1992). New graduates in critical care: How long do they stay? *Critical Care Nurse, 12*(8), 74–79.

Hughes, L. (1987). Employment of new graduates: Implications for critical nursing practice. *Focus on Critical Care, 14*(4), 9–15.

Lindy, C. N., & Reiter, P. (2006). The financial impact of staff development. *Journal of Continuing Education in Nursing, 37*(3), 121–127.

Messmer, P. R., Abelleira, A., & Erb, P. S. (1995). Code 50: An orientation matrix to track orientation cost. *Journal of Nursing Staff Development, 11*(5), 261–264.

Using NDNQI's RN Satisfaction Survey Results to Track Satisfaction with Appropriateness of Patient Assignments

Kim Maryniak, RNC, BN, MSN
Professional Development Coordinator
Kmaryniak@yumaregional.org

Yuma Regional Medical Center

Editor's Pick

INSIGHTS & IDEAS FROM THIS FACILITY

Improved satisfaction with patient assignments was based on identifying and addressing unit-specific issues. Examples included adding more staff and training in the care of overflow patient populations.

Facility and Unit Summary

Facility	Yuma Regional Medical Center (YRMC)—Yuma, Arizona **http://www.yumaregional.org**
Facility setting	Geographically located to serve the southwestern portion of Arizona, the southeastern portion of California, and the northern tip of Mexico, and the sole community hospital provider for Yuma City and Yuma County
Teaching status	Nonteaching
Ownership status	Not-for-profit community hospital
Community demographics	Third fastest growing area in the country for the period 1990–2006; population of county served by YRMC: • 50.5% Hispanic or Latino (many first- or second-generation U.S. citizens) • 44% non-Hispanic white; • Remainder made up of Asians, blacks, other non-Hispanic groups • Approximately 16% of population of service area over 65 years.
Hospital-staffed beds	333 beds
Case mix index (CMI)	1.07
Indicators used	RN Satisfaction Survey
System or units improved	3 West Surgical Pediatric–Women's Gynecological Unit
Indicator improved	Patient Assignment Was Appropriate
QI documents used	NDNQI RN Survey Reports
Time frame of QI experience	2004–2007
NDNQI® participation	Since 2003
Magnet™ status	Applying for Magnet recognition
Governance model	Shared Governance

Awards and recognition

- Institute for Healthcare Improvement Mentor Site (for wound, ostomy, and pressure ulcer prevention)—2007
- Professional Research Consultants Top Performer Award—2007
- American Diabetes Association Education Recognition Certificate—2007
- Partners in Trauma Award from Banner—2006
- AARP Best Employers Program—2006
- Overall Winner, Southwest Arizona Human Resource Association Great Place to Work—2006
- Arizona Society for Human Resources Management State
- Council Workforce Diversity—2006
- American Society for Healthcare Engineering (ASHE) recognition for cutting the hospital's energy use per square foot (part of the ASHE Energy Efficiency Commitment Initiative)—2006

UNIT PROFILES

3 West

Internal name

3 West (Surgical)

Size and type

3 West is a 52-bed inpatient orthopedic surgical unit

Staff summary

- Resource coordinators, functioning in the charge nurse role
- Registered nurses (RNs), as lead bedside caregivers
- Clinical associates (nursing assistants), working with RNs on team
- Business associates (unit clerks), providing clerical support and order processing
- Team associates, providing environmental services and some assistance with patient transfers
- Unit-based educators
- Patient attendants, providing sitter assistance for patients with high risk of falls

Organizational structure

Unit director, Unit educator, Resource coordinators, Bedside and support staff

WCU

Internal name	WCU (Women and Children's Unit)
Size and type	23-bed combined pediatric and women's gynecological surgery unit, with overflow from post-partum and women's medical patients and specializing in pediatrics and women's gynecological surgery
Staff summary:	• Resource coordinators, functioning in the charge nurse role • RNs serving as lead bedside caregivers • Clinical associates (nursing assistants), working with RNs on team • Business associates (unit clerks), providing clerical support and order processing • Team associates, providing environmental services and some assistance with patient transfers • Unit-based educators
Organizational structure	Unit director, Unit educator, Resource coordinators, Bedside and support staff

	3 West (Surgical)	WCU (Medical)
Staffing (full-time employees—FTEs)		
Resource coordinator	4.00	3.60
Registered nurses	50.50	11.90
Clinical associates	23.35	3.60
Business associates	6.13	4.20
Team associates	8.95	3.60
Patient attendants	3.75	0.00
Educators	1.00	1.00
Skill mix	64% RN	70% RN
% ADN	67	64
% BSN	20	36
% Certified	18	21
Nurse–patient ratio (NHPPD)	1:5 to 1:6	1:4 to 1:6

Using NDNQI's RN Satisfaction Survey Results to Track Satisfaction with Appropriateness of Patient Assignments

Kim Maryniak, RNC, BN, MSN

Yuma Regional Medical Center

Introductory Summary

Yuma Regional Medical Center (YRMC) is a 333-bed, acute-care, nonprofit, community-based hospital that provides healthcare services for Yuma, Arizona, and the surrounding community. The hospital facility is geographically located to serve the southwestern portion of Arizona, the southeastern portion of California, and the northern tip of Mexico. The city of Yuma is located along Interstate 8 and the Colorado River. The Colorado River is a glittering ribbon of water that seems totally out of place in the middle of the Sonoran desert in which Yuma County is located. Water from the river supports the agricultural, tourist, and residential activities in the area.

Healthcare services at YRMC are based on patient needs; special consideration is given to growth and developmental milestones for specialized-age populations and to cultural backgrounds, including ethnicity and language needs. The remote location of YRMC presents unique challenges. These challenges guide both the philosophy and the strategic initiatives of the organization in the mission of quality patient care. The YRMC team commits itself to excellence in patient care at every level of service. As the regional referral center, healthcare professionals provide a diverse range of services to a diverse patient population. The YRMC's 13-member community board offers guidance for strategic planning, governance, and direction of the hospital. A primary goal of the hospital is cost-effective access to programs, services, and medical expertise in Yuma and the remote surrounding areas.

The culture at Yuma Regional Medical Center is dynamic, relationship-oriented, and multidisciplinary. Nursing has strived to maintain the enthusiasm and dedication that conveys a center for excellence. The organization has been engaged in a Journey to Excellence program for many years and continues to produce an environment that supports growth, innovation, education, and evidence-based practice.

In preparation for the 2005 fiscal year, nurse leadership at YRMC examined evidence for the impact of nurse staffing. One example was using recommendations from *The Journal of the American Medical Association* (Aiken, 2002), which identified the following concerns: (1)There are consistent reports that nurse staffing levels are inadequate to provide safe and effective care. (2) Nursing staff shortages are major impediments to the provision of high-quality hospital care. (3) Nursing workloads are unrealistic. (4) Of hospital nurses, 40% have burnout levels that exceed norms for healthcare workers. (5) Job dissatisfaction among nurses is four times the average for all U.S. workers. (6) One out of every five hospital nurses plans to leave his or her current job within 1 year. The article concluded that registered nurse staffing has a significant impact on avoidable deaths in hospitals. It also suggested that nurse staffing levels are primary recruitment and retention tools, as they reduce the potential for burnout and dissatisfaction on the job.

Another consideration was the Institute of Medicine (IOM) report (Morrissey, 2003), which recommended the following: "Facilities should incorporate some excess nurse capacity into each shift to accommodate unanticipated increases in workload." The report also called for "giving nurses the authority to halt admissions to their units when they determine that staffing is inadequate to take any new patients." The IOM report went on to say that "hospitals must find ways to scale back the workload of their staff nurses, send them off to training sessions more often, provide continuing educating opportunities, and avoid using agencies for fill-in nurses to maintain patient safety."

Use of this evidence was discussed with staff and presented in a white paper for justification of additional nursing FTEs during FY 2004–2005. This paper was written by two nursing directors, in collaboration with the nurse leadership group (Moore & Fike, 2004).

During the same period, YRMC was beginning to develop the Excellence in Nursing program, to identify excellence and reward nurses. Patricia Benner's Novice to Expert theory (Benner, 2001) was distinguished as being suited for the culture at YRMC. Numerous subgroups were developed with many bedside nurses and members of nurse leadership to formulate new job descriptions based on Benner's theory. Thus, nurses have been identified as novice/advanced beginner, competent, proficient, and expert. In addition, the American Association of Critical Care Nurses (AACN) Synergy Model (Reed, 2008) had been used in the Intensive Care Unit for a few years. In examining the components of this model, the subgroups agreed that this model better described nursing than the previous job descriptions had. The categories of advocacy/moral agency, caring practices, collaboration, systems thinking, response to diversity, clinical inquiry, and facilitation of learning were adopted to describe nursing skills, knowledge, and application at YRMC.

Two units at YRMC have shown sustained improvement in the percentage of RNs who believe their patient assignments are appropriate. Different strategies, adapted to unit conditions, have been used to promote satisfaction with patient assignments.

Data on satisfaction with patient assignments came from the NDNQI RN Satisfaction Surveys, conducted at YRMC since 2005. While the initial YRMC response rate was above the national average, YRMC nursing leaders wanted to hear from every nurse to ensure that the survey portrayed significant representation of different RN perspectives. The YRMC survey committee distributed a letter to all RNs to promote participation in the survey as part of the facility's Journey to Excellence. RNs, in turn, were eager to let their voices be heard. In the 2007 survey, 97% of YRMC's direct care RNs responded to the survey.

3 West Surgical

The goal of the surgical unit 3 West, a 52-bed inpatient unit, is to provide high-quality care to adult patients undergoing diagnostic testing or surgical intervention, recovering from an illness or posttrauma treatment, or undergoing radiation oncology therapy. For patients whose health may not improve, the goal is to provide care with dignity, offering support to the patient and family as needed. Generally, a patient is considered a candidate for admission if they are 15 years of age or older; experience an acute illness or potentially acute illness, trauma, other surgical condition, or potential surgical condition; or experience exacerbation of a chronic condition, affecting one or more body systems. The unit also specializes in orthopedic surgery.

Patient Assignment on 3 West

In 2005, the RN survey data showed that RNs on 3 West rated "Patient assignment was appropriate" at 3.96 on a scale of 1 to 6, with 1 representing "strongly disagree" and 6 representing "strongly agree." In speaking with staff on the unit interviewers identified several factors as concerns with patient assignments. In particular, RNs were displeased with how patient load was affected by scheduled surgeries, as well as the amount of time required for admissions, discharges, and transfers.

Information from a variety of sources that could help frame the problem was assessed. The information included data from NDNQI; number of admissions, discharges, and transfers; medication volume; patient acuity; and surgery volume. The results were presented and discussed at focused meetings with the unit director, eight senior nurses, two resource coordinators, and four new graduates. The information was then reviewed with the 3 West leadership group at a retreat. The leadership group developed a draft action plan that the director took to the 3 West Unit Leadership Council. The council reviewed the draft workload management plan, voted on it, and prioritized what should be implemented on a trial basis.

Four strategies were implemented. First, new guidelines were developed for patient assignments that took into account RN skill (based on RN experience), patient acuity, and projected surgery volume. Second, strategies were formulated for partnering senior staff with new graduate nurses or junior staff. Third, on shifts with scheduled higher census of acute surgeries, such as orthopedic surgeries, additional RNs were to be added. Fourth, an admission, discharge, transfer (ADT) nurse was made available to 3 West during times of high patient acuity and turnover to assist with ADTs. The justification for the extra FTEs was documented in a policy paper written by the nursing directors in the medical/surgical division (Moore & Fike, 2004). Sign-up lists for the ADT role, as well as the use of seasonal staff, helped to increase satisfaction with patient assignments.

FIGURE 1.
RN Satisfaction with Patient Assignment, 3 West

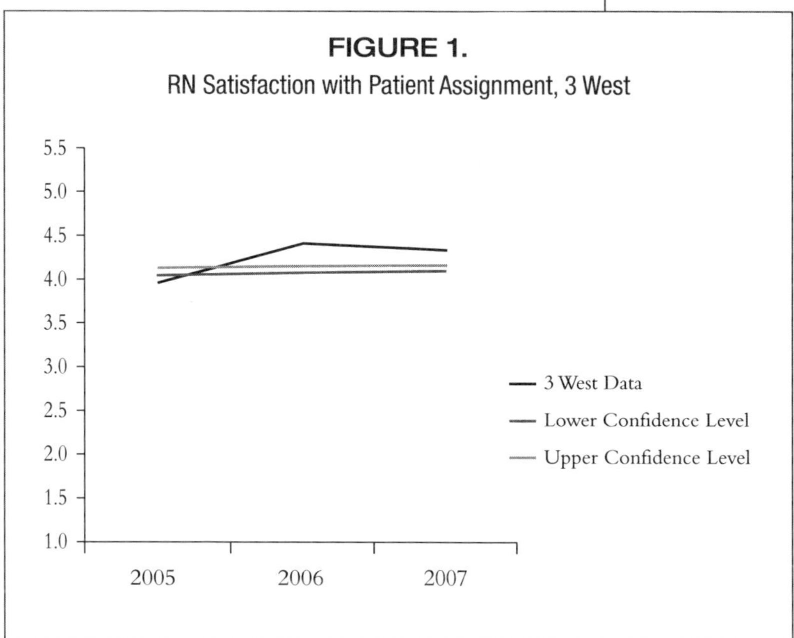

The results (see Figure 1) showed an improvement in the question on patient assignments, from 3.96 in 2005 to 4.38 in 2006, and remaining at the same level in the 2007 survey (4.35). In 2007, the agreement with "Patient assignment was appropriate" on 3 West was near the NDNQI upper quartile cut point of 4.48, the score achieved by the top 25 percent of surgical units. In sum, 3 West RNs' agreement with the statement that their patient assignment was appropriate was above the national norm in both 2006 and 2007.

The additional FTEs raised total nursing hours per patient day on 3 West from 7.04 in 2005 to 7.78 in 2007. These staffing levels were lower than the NDNQI means for surgical units of 300- to 399-bed hospitals (8.46 in 2005 and 8.41 in 2007). However, they reflect an improvement in nursing hours since 2005.

The RN survey results on appropriate assignment, in conjunction with the NDNQI comparison data for nursing hours per patient day, were used to support the 2009 budget request for 3 West to maintain the additional staff to work with fluctuating acuity and to manage admissions, discharges, and transfers. Data have been collected and reviewed to distribute the extra staff during peak hours and shifts, and to assign a workload value for ADTs.

Women and Children's Unit

The goal of the Women and Children's Unit (WCU) is to provide quality health care directed toward meeting the physiological, psychological, and spiritual needs of patients. The unit is a 24-bed unit consisting of all private rooms, isolation rooms, and a playroom. There is a Sick Child Care Center located on the unit, which provides care to ill children of staff at YRMC in order to allow the employees to work. The WCU specializes in pediatric patients and gynecological surgery patients. This unit can be used as an overflow area for post-partum and women's medical patients, when those units have surpassed capacity.

The 2005 NDNQI RN Satisfaction Survey score on "Patient assignment was appropriate" was 4.17 for the staff of the WCU, below the national average for medical units (4.61). As staff input showed, the main factor that affected the RN satisfaction was the level of comfort in caring for overflow patient populations. Because of the increase in deliveries at YRMC during 2004–2005, the volume of overflow post-partum patients grew. This not only included post-partum couplets (including mothers and babies), but also included women patients with fetal demise. The nurses on the unit were competent to expert in caring for pediatric and women's surgical patients. However, nursing leaders who gathered information on the reasons for dissatisfaction with staffing levels found that WCU RNs did not feel they had the education or experience needed to care competently for the post-partum population.

In order to meet the needs of the staff, collaboration was required between the directors and educators of the departments of the Division of Women and Children Services: the WCU; the Neonatal Intensive Care Unit (NICU); and Labor, Delivery, Recovery, and Post-Partum (LDRP). As a result, didactic classes that were offered to LDRP and NICU staff also were offered to RNs in the Women and Children's Unit. In addition, in recognition of the skilled expertise of LDRP staff in working with families with fetal demise, it was determined that placement of these patients should remain in LDRP.

The Division of Women and Children Services holds an annual skills fair. Staff from WCU were assigned not only to their usual stations, but also to stations that related to post-partum care and neonates. These included teachings on various topics, such as fetal demise, neonatal abnormalities, substance abuse infants, developmental care, breastfeeding, and post-partum/newborn care.

Figure 2 shows the increase in satisfaction with patient assignments on the WCU from 4.17 in 2005 to 4.87 in 2006. Satisfaction with patient assignments continued to grow in 2007 to 5.24, placing the WCU among the top 25% of all medical units on this measure (above the NDNQI top quartile cut point of 5.03). Thus by 2007, RN satisfaction with patient assignments in the WCU was in the top 25% of all pediatric units in the country participating in the NDNQI RN Satisfaction Survey.

Greater levels of WCU staff agreement with "Patient assignment was appropriate" occurred with the addition of staff to the unit. Total nursing hours per patient day on the WCU was 8.36 in 2005 and 10.93 in 2007. Although these levels were below the NDNQI national mean for pediatric/medical units of 300- to 399-bed hospitals, they represent a meaningful increase in nursing hours per patient day for WCU.

The success of the shared divisional skills fair has led to its being offered every year, with topics centering on new evidence-based information and high-risk, low-volume areas. Continued didactics are provided, and the organization also participates in an online site for available continuing education courses.

Conclusion and Implications

Evidence-based practice has been an important component of the Journey to Excellence program at Yuma Regional Medical Center. In addition to using the NDNQI survey and comparison data, the implications of appropriate nurse staffing at YRMC have been and continue to be demonstrated in its nursing satisfaction scores. By using the evidence from reference sources, nursing FTEs and assignments can be made appropriately (Aiken, 2002; Morrissey, 2003). Adopting and incorporating both Benner's Novice to Expert theory (2001) and Reed's AACN Synergy Model (Reed, 2008) also helped YRMC to identify the strengths, diversity, and significance of the impact of nurses to quality patient care. This experience has also demonstrated the need for life-long education and professional development, ongoing processes along the continuum of nursing careers (Ridge, 2005).

The improvements made in both the surgical unit 3 West and the Women and Children's Unit demonstrate that different and distinct courses of action were employed. In addition to increased nurse staffing levels, increased satisfaction with the appropriateness of patient satisfaction was based on different courses of action responsive to each unit's perceived problems. It is vital to use shared governance and gather input from those involved to identify and meet the specific needs of RNs on different units. Solutions vary from situation to situation, along with the diverse and unique qualities of both staff and patient populations. Use of the NDNQI RN Satisfaction Survey assists in recognizing not only areas requiring improvement, but also areas deserving merit. The NDNQI survey is just one tool utilized in the continuous development and progression toward providing quality care in an environment of excellence.

FIGURE 2.
RN Satisfaction with Patient Assignment, WCU

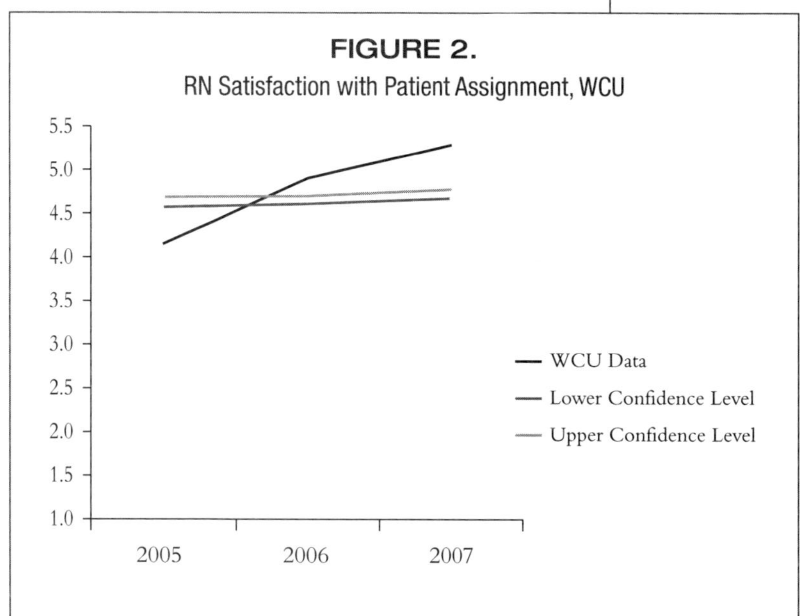

References

Aiken, L. (2002). Hospital nurse staffing and patient mortality, nurse burnout, and job dissatisfaction. *Journal of the American Medical Association, 288*(16), 1987–1993.

Benner, P. (2001). *From novice to expert: Excellence and power in clinical nursing practice* (Commemorative edition). Reading/Menlo Park: Addison-Wesley.

Moore, M., & Fike, R. (2004). *Nursing FTEs for budget year 2004–2005* (White Paper). Yuma Regional Medical Center, Yuma, AZ.

Morrissey, J. (2003). Quality vs. quantity; IOM report; Hospitals must cut back workload and hours of nurses to maintain patient safety. *Modern Healthcare, 33*(45), 8, 11.

Reed, K. (2008). The AACN Synergy Model for patient care: A nursing model as a force of magnetism. *Nursing Economics, 26*(1), 17–25.

Ridge, R. (2005). A dynamic duo: Staff development, orientation, and you. *Nursing Management, 36*(7).

Hospital Acquired Pressure Ulcers

Defined:

A pressure ulcer is any lesion caused by **unrelieved pressure** resulting in damage of underlying tissue. They may be located over bony prominences or skin surfaces subject to excess pressure such as under a medical device/equipment. They are staged according to the extent of observable tissue damage. The nurse observer should be able to distinguish a pressure ulcer from other types of wounds and skin conditions (e.g., venous or arterial ulcers, diabetic foot ulcers, yeast infections, maceration, perineal dermatitis, skin tears, or operating room-acquired cautery burns). Count the number of pressure ulcers on each patient, whether acquired since admission to your facility or acquired before admission.

Hospital acquired refers to new ulcer(s) developed **after** admission to a facility, also termed nosocomial or facility acquired. The hospital admission assessment should be reviewed for the presence of ulcers. If there is no documentation that the ulcer was present on admission, then the ulcer(s) should be counted as hospital acquired.

Formulas:

Total Pressure Ulcer Prevalence: Prevalence Number of patients with Ulcers/ Number of patients in survey

Hospital Acquired Pressure Ulcer: Prevalence Number of Patients with Hospital Acquired Ulcers/Number of Patients in Survey

Point-of-Care Education Reduces Pressure Ulcer Rates in the ICU

Susan Reeder, RN, MS CWCN
Burn/Wound Resource Nurse
REEDES@mmc.org

Nicole Manchester, RN, MS, CCRN
Clinical Nurse Leader

Sonja Orff-Ney, RN, MS
Clinical Nurse Leader

Denise Dende, BA, MFA
Center for Nursing Research and Quality Outcomes

Carole Parisien, MSN, RN
Nursing Analyst, Center for Nursing Research and Quality Outcomes

Maine Medical Center

Editor's Pick

INSIGHTS & IDEAS FROM THIS FACILITY

Comprehensive pressure ulcer prevention program includes unit-based skin teams that provide point-of-care education on skin maintenance to staff nurses.

Facility and Unit Summary

Facility	Maine Medical Center (MMC)—Portland, Maine **http://www.mmc.org**
Facility setting	The largest hospital in Maine, MMC is a community-based, six-campus, acute care teaching hospital located in suburban southern Maine, serving 31,000 inpatients and 68,000 outpatients every year. Services feature cardiac services (including open heart surgery), orthopedics, and neurosurgery, pediatrics, gynecology, and Maine's only kidney and pancreas transplant program, Level I trauma center, Level III neonatal nursery, and academic medical center.
Teaching status	Teaching hospital (academic affiliations with seven colleges for nursing education; offers residency and fellowship programs in over 18 specialty areas)
Ownership status	Private nonprofit
Community demographics	Service population is 230,000 in the Greater Portland area. Predominantly Caucasian (96.6% white) and multiethnic with: • 1.6% Black • 0.1% American Indian • 0.4% Hispanic • 0.9% Asian • 0.4% other Approximately 16% of the service area population is over age 65.
Hospital-staffed beds	499
Case mix index (CMI)	1.98
Indicators used	All available indicators
System or unit improved	Unit improvement (cardiothoracic ICU, special care unit for adult med/surg, pediatric patients)
Indicators improved	Hospital acquired pressure ulcers
QI documents used	Monthly nursing balanced scorecard with NDNQI quarterly benchmarks
NDNQI® participation	Since 2003
Time frame of QI experience	2006–2007
Magnet™ status	Magnet designation May 2006

Awards and recognition	• Ranked #41 in the nation for Gynecology Care (U.S. News and World Report)—2008 • Ranked #45 for Orthopedic Care and #50 for Heart Attack Care (U.S. News & World Report)—2007 • Top 100 "Most Wired" Hospitals and Top 25 "Most Wireless" Hospitals —2006 • Ranked #4 on Consumer's Digest "50 Exceptional U.S. Hospitals"—2005 • Top 5% in nation for Cardiology Services and Joint Replacement (Health Grades)—2005

UNIT PROFILES

CTICU

Internal name	CTICU (Cardiothoracic Intensive Care Unit)
Size and type	4-bed cardiothoracic surgery intensive care unit
Staff summary	• Education: 12% diploma; 21% AD; 60% BSN; 7% MSN • 52.17% full-time; 26.09% part-time; 21.74% per diem • 19% of RNs with national certification in specialty area
Skill mix	83.5% RNs; 14.5% CNAs
Nurse-patient ratio (NHPPD)	21.63
Organizational structure	Nursing director, Nurse manager, Staff (charge nurse, unit-based educator, clinical nurse leader)

SCU

Internal name	SCU (Special Care Unit)
Size and type	32-bed medical/surgical adult and pediatric special care unit
Staff summary	• Education: 6% diploma; 20% AD; 67% BSN; 6% MSN • 53.33% full-time; 28.15% part-time; 18.52% per diem • 28% of RNs with national certification in specialty area
Skill mix	77.14% RNs; 17.15% CNAs; 3.43% NUSs
Nurse-patient ratio (NHPPD)	19.86
Organizational structure	Nursing director, Nurse manager, Staff (charge nurse, unit-based educator, clinical nurse leader, unit coordinator)

Point-of-Care Education Reduces Pressure Ulcer Rates in the ICU

Susan Reeder, RN, MS, CWCN
Nicole Manchester, RN, MS, CCRN
Sonja Orff-Ney, RN, MS
Denise Dende, BA, MFA
Carole Parisien, MSN, RN

Maine Medical Center

Introductory Summary

The Special Care Unit (SCU) and Cardiothoracic Intensive Care Unit (CTICU) at Maine Medical Center (MMC) demonstrated hospital acquired pressure ulcer (HAPU) rates above the national mean rates for adult critical care units for five out of six quarters between Q1-06 and Q4-07 based on the National Database of Nursing Quality Indicators® (NDNQI). A multipronged approach was undertaken, which featured three interventions implemented simultaneously. The interventions consisted of skin rounds, participation in a Volunteer Hospital Association (VHA) pressure ulcer prevention program, and point-of-care education. The most prominent and successful intervention was "skin rounds," undertaken initially by the critical care clinical nurse leaders (CNLs) and the critical care certified wound care nurse (CWCN) to create discussion and point-of-care education for staff nurses on pressure ulcer identification and prevention. Over time, the skin rounds project grew to include additional RN staff, support staff, respiratory and physical therapists, nutritional services, patients, and families.

Following the above intervention, HAPU rates for adult critical care fell below the NDNQI mean for Adult Critical Care for the Q3/Q4-07. Success has been measured by the acceptance of skin rounds as a routine weekly occurrence, increased staff participation in rounds, and more appropriate use of products, particularly in the areas of incontinence care and moisture management.

Facility at a Glance

Maine Medical Center is a 606-bed tertiary-care center serving northern New England, with 400 to 499 staffed beds. MMC provides comprehensive inpatient services in all medical specialties and is the largest teaching hospital in Maine, as well as being recognized as the only Level I Trauma Center in Maine. The hospital provides services and specialties unavailable elsewhere in Maine or, often, in northern New England. MMC received Magnet™ recognition for excellence in nursing service in 2006. MMC also is proud to be recognized nationally for cardiovascular surgical care, gynecology, and orthopedics.

MMC has several critical care units with a diverse mix of patients. The CTICU is a 14-bed cardiothoracic surgery intensive care unit with an average daily census of nine critically ill adult patients requiring postoperative recovery from open heart surgery, surgical patients requiring cardiopulmonary bypass, as well as thoracic and vascular surgery patients requiring critical care. The SCU is a 32-bed medical/surgical adult and pediatric special care unit with an average daily census of 29 critically ill patients. The SCU is divided into three separate sections, two 10-bed sections and one 12-bed section. The unit provides 24-hour continuous monitoring and specialized nursing care to medical, surgical, trauma, neurological, transplant, burn, and pediatric cardiac surgical patients, and critically ill infants and children.

NDNQI Start-Up Considerations

Maine Medical Center has been collecting HAPU data monthly since 1994. One of the challenges experienced over the years is that while pressure ulcer data were collected, the data were not readily available to staff in a timely fashion and were distributed via posters and e-mail. Initially the data entry process was time consuming, and results were not available for 3 to 5 weeks after data collection. In 2006, raw pressure ulcer data began to be entered on a shared drive on an Excel spreadsheet in the hospital computer system, which was accessible to all staff. The time from when data are collected to when they are able to be viewed was reduced to less than 1 week.

Maine Medical Center began submitting data to NDNQI in the spring of 2003. By 2005–2006, NDNQI pressure ulcer data, as well as the results of internal pressure ulcer data collection, were readily available to staff in an electronic format. Data trends along with benchmark data from NDNQI were displayed electronically on a table referred to as the scorecard. Staff have access to both the scorecard and unit raw data. Access to unit raw data via the Excel format enables staff to see details such as demographic data (age, gender, hospital day), risk assessment, interventions, and the stage and location of ulcers found and on which unit the ulcers originated. Identifying specific trends enables staff to better tailor future pressure ulcer interventions. The NDNQI pressure ulcer data allowed MMC staff to compare results to other hospitals the same size and to raise MMC's standards on pressure ulcer prevention.

Pressure Ulcer Program

For the past 14 years, Maine Medical Center has had an organized, systematic approach to pressure ulcer identification and data collection. Over the past 5 to 8 years, increased attention and resources have been allocated to developing a hospitalwide pressure ulcer prevention program. Nursing representatives from each unit, including registered nurses and nursing assistants, were designated as the skin team representatives. Skin team representatives were trained by the wound, ostomy, and continence nurse (WOCN) team. Skin team training included education on pressure ulcer staging (including an inter-rater reliability process), the data collection process, and basic prevention strategies. The skin team met monthly to review data (both internal data and comparison data from NDNQI), discuss difficult cases and determine prevention interventions, review new products, and network with each other. After the meetings, staff returned to their units to collect pressure ulcer data, which included a head-to-toe evaluation of all patients on each unit. The program continued to grow under the support and leadership of the chief nursing officer and nursing directors, who ensure that staff have time away from direct patient care duties to participate.

Interventions

Due to increasing HAPU rates in 2006, the clinical nurse leaders in the CTICU and the SCU were charged by the chief nursing officer with the task of formulating a strategic plan to address the increasing pressure ulcer rates.

The CNLs first worked separately with the certified wound care nurse in order to identify and address issues that were specific to their individual patient populations. Early interventions included focusing on operating room tables, decreasing the amount of bed linen used under patients, developing a resource manual to help with product choices for treatment and prevention of pressure ulcer/wounds, stocking the unit with hydrocolloids and barrier sprays to prevent delays in obtaining the products, and creating a skin care competency or educational self-study module for both the bedside nurse and support staff. All of these interventions helped engage and empower the staff.

Following the implementation of the interventions noted above, the CNLs and the CWCN decided to work collaboratively to synergize efforts and achieve common goals. This multipronged approach featured three interventions that were implemented simultaneously: skin rounds, participation in the Voluntary Hospital Association program, and point-of-care education.

Skin Rounds

Skin rounds was the leading intervention in the multipronged approach that began in June 2007. The major focus of skin rounds was to provide point-of-care education to the bedside nurse. It was an opportunity to assess each patient along with the nurse caring for the patient, formulate a plan of care together, and aid in communication of that plan. Education was given at the bedside so direct care providers and family members had the opportunity to participate. Knowing that it is difficult for staff to attend a class, education was instead incorporated into the patient's daily care. One-on-one teaching was provided during rounds. For example, staff did not always know how to best assess incontinence issues, both with fecal incontinence prevention and the use of skin barrier products. If patients were having issues with fecal incontinence, discussion was centered on prevention of diarrhea, including topics such as discontinuation of sorbitol-containing liquid medications, early identification and treatment of infectious diarrhea, use of antidiarrheal medication when appropriate, fecal containment systems, and barrier cream products. Upon learning that most of the patients had problems with incontinence, additional education was provided on identifying ulcers due to moisture (incontinence-associated dermatitis) as opposed to ulcers due to pressure. Too many skin barrier products also were found in the patient's bedside table in the rooms. This led to inconsistent use of products and, in some cases, less-effective products being used.

Moisture was the second major clinical problem encountered. Many of the ICU patients were edematous and immobile, making it difficult to keep their skin clean and dry. During skin rounds, the CWCN and CNL consulted with staff and helped increase the use of absorptive dressings, barrier film spray, and application of antifungal powders to skin folds. For patients with moisture problems, reusable bed pads were replaced with absorptive breathable disposable pads, which not only performed better, but reduced wrinkles and multiple layers of linen under the patient. Low air loss beds were recommended for immobile patients with severe moisture problems.

By rounding on each patient, staff were challenged to increase turning schedules of immobile, unstable patients. The CNL, CWCN, and bedside nurse, working as a team, would reposition patients during rounds. During this time, the CNL and CWCN would role model pressure-reduction techniques, demonstrating that it could be done safely. Most patients were able to tolerate at least small changes in position. Role modeling and mentoring during skin rounds also were responsive to the nurses' immediate needs to care for the patient.

The plan of care was posted in each patient's room for staff unable to attend rounds, and for patients and families. The plan posted in the room provided an opportunity to share information (see the process and documentation sheet in Figure 1). In an effort to include the night and weekend staff, skin rounds also were also performed during those times, although not as regularly.

The initial intent of the intervention was to round on

FIGURE 1.

Plan of Care: Skin Rounds Process and Documentation

Objectives of Skin Rounds:

- To create change in the current work environment that reflects skin assessment/awareness as a shared responsibility among all disciplines.
- To formulate a rescue plan so that all patients who can't reposition themselves effectively will be repositioned every two hours or more frequently as needed.
- To increase awareness of patients at risk for skin breakdown and reduce pressure ulcer rates.
- To demonstrate through role modeling adequate documentation and turning of the assigned patient by both the RN and the CNA.
- To foster an environment that empowers staff to share responsibility, communicate, and collaborate.

Interventions During Skin Rounds:

- CWCN's and CNL's lead weekly rounds in CTICU and SCU.
- Education was provided to staff, patients, and family members at the bedside.
- Patients with Braden Score <19 receive full skin assessment.
- A plan of care is created involving the input of the multidisciplinary team (nurse, support staff, respiratory therapy, rehab medicine, nutritional services, and other departments).
- The plan of care is posted in each patient's room to share with staff, patient, and family.
- Preventive measures and wound care are implemented by the rounding team (repositioning, moisture management, dressing changes).

The written plan of care is electronically updated to reflect the new skin care plan.

Skin Care Rounds

Date: ____________________

Present: ____________________

Skin breakdown documented before today? ____________ Braden Scale: ________

Pressure Ulcer Risk Interventions

___ Manage moisture, nutrition, and friction & shear
___ Protect heels
___ Frequent turning
___ Supplement with small shifts
___ Use pressure-relieving surface (Kinair or Bari Maxx)
___ Schedule turning
___ Other: ____________________

Skin Assessment:

1. Back of head
2. Right ear
3. Left ear
4. Right scapular
5. Left scapular
6. Right elbow
7. Left elbow
8. Vertebra (upper-mid)
9. Sacrum
10. Coccyx
11. Right buttock
12. Left buttock
13. Right iliac crest
14. Left iliac crest
15. Right trochanter (hip)
16. Left trochanter (hip)
17. Right ischial tuberosity
18. Left ischial tuberosity
19. Right thigh
20. Left thigh
21. Right knee
22. Left knee
23. Right lower leg
24. Left lower leg
25. Right ankle (inner/outer)
26. Left ankle (inner/outer)
27. Right heel
28. Left heel
29. Right toe(s)
30. Left toe(s)
31. Other (specify)

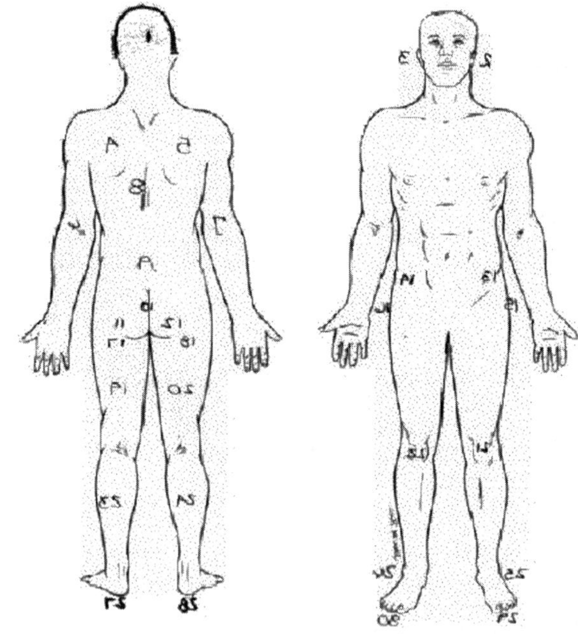

Discussed with ____________________
(RN responsible to implement plan/changes)

New Plan:

Turn patient Q 2 hours and document in eCare

all intensive care unit (ICU) patients in each 10-bed section weekly. However, because the time required for these educational rounds was extensive, only one section per week was feasible (approximately 10 to 12 patients).

VHA Project

The second intervention undertaken in the multipronged approach was the participation of MMC in the Voluntary Hospital Association of New England's skin care project during the fall of 2007. The critical care team participated in this initiative. The focus of the initiative was on tests of small changes. The initiative chosen for the project included evaluation of increased routine repositioning or turning of patients and turning documentation. Results showed that patients were being repositioned every 2 hours, but the documentation was inconsistent, because there were multiple options for charting turns in the electronic record. Due to the inability to reprogram the electronic system, a separate paper document was created. Ultimately this method of documentation was not successful, as it took too much time away from patient care. While this test of change ultimately was not sustainable for staff, it provided insight into system issues.

Point-of-Care Education

The third element in the multipronged approach carried out during the intervention period was education. Education was provided via several avenues. Training for RN and CNA staff was completed using self-study packets (2006 and 2007), classes were provided by the WOCN nurses, informal education occurred at the bedside above and beyond rounds, and skin care was included during precepting of new nursing orientees. Content included pressure ulcer identification; moisture versus pressure lesions; risk assessment; staging; prevention interventions, especially moisture management and pressure reduction; incontinence care; and nutrition interventions. The RN representatives to the skin care committee completed the NDNQI Pressure Ulcer Assessment tutorial in February 2008.

FIGURE 2.
HAPU Rates (%) in SCU and CTICU as compared to NDNQI during 2006 (pre-intervention) and 2007 (post-intervention)

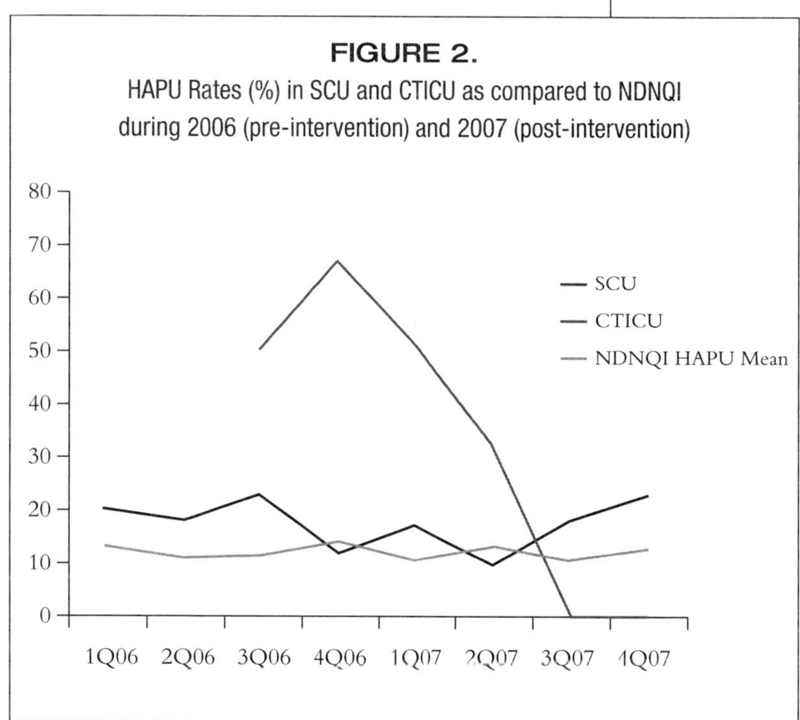

Data Summary and Outcomes

Hospital acquired pressure ulcer rates in the SCU and CTICU were above the mean HAPU NDNQI critical care rates for hospitals with 400 to 499 staff beds for most of 2006 and half of 2007. CTICU HAPU rates peaked during the fourth quarter of 2006 at 66.67%. When compared with the lowest rate for the CTICU—fourth quarter of 2007 (0.00%)—this represented a 100% decrease in HAPU rates in the CTICU (see Figure 2). The HAPU rates for the SCU varied over time, being above the national NDNQI rate one quarter and below it the next.

Conclusions and Implications

Nursing staff now have a better understanding for the treatment and prevention of pressure ulcers. There is less waste of supplies and more consistency in treatment. Pressure ulcer rates have decreased and continue to improve. Through the sharing of the NDNQI data, staff can see how the pressure ulcer rates in their units compare to peer units across the United States. NDNQI data provide staff with valuable information to chart their progress toward the goal of zero pressure ulcers. Achieving multidisciplinary success includes support staff reciting the correct treatment plan, orientation for the new nurse, physical therapists' noticing a patients buttock is appearing red and alerting the skin team, respiratory therapy assisting the bedside nurse to get the patient back to bed, and the therapist suggesting moving the oxygen saturation probe to the opposite ear to prevent skin breakdown.

Long before the new Medicare policies on reimbursement for HAPUs were instituted, MMC had a target of zero pressure ulcers as an important part of quality care. The belief that pressure ulcers were an unavoidable consequence of being critically ill has changed. Now HAPUs are viewed as "never events," or consequences that should never happen.

Challenges with documentation of pressure ulcers and skin care plans continue, since the electronic documentation system does not have one place for clear communication. The skin care team approach of going from patient to patient with nursing staff gave staff an opportunity to participate in the evaluation and treatment plan for the patient. Now it is common practice for the bedside nurse to have implemented moisture management techniques and repositioning schedules even for the sickest patients.

If a patient does develop a hospital acquired pressure ulcer, the team, including nurses, the CWCN, physicians, the therapist, and dieticians, are alerted right away and a new plan of care is posted in the room. Since starting skin rounds, staff are more likely to consult with the CWCN for minor skin problems, including blanchable erythema, for suggestions on repositioning devices that could cause pressure, and for friction and shear management before the skin is broken. Prior to this project, the CWCN was often consulted after the patient's skin had become compromised. Family members can generate a consult to the CWCN by verbal request during skin rounds or through communication with the bedside nurse or unit secretary.

Staff now have a better understanding of the prevention and treatment of pressure ulcers. Standardization of barrier products led to their more consistent use. An algorithm was developed for fecal containment devices, and now the equipment is stored in the unit.

The CNLs and staff have become resources to other areas of the hospital who want to begin their own "skin rounds" project. The data collection tool is being used in several patient care areas. New nurse orientees frequently attend skin rounds in the critical care areas to observe and learn about skin care. It is important to recognize that managing skin integrity in a vulnerable and sick population is complex. There are many elements to consider, and it is critical to create a synergy among nursing staff to devise a plan that is comprehensive, effective, and efficient. Skin rounds continue to take place weekly in one section of critical care and focus on interventions to prevent pressure, moisture, friction, or sheer from causing areas of potential breakdown.

Hospital acquired pressure ulcer rates continue to be monitored. Future plans include analysis of patient variables for patients who developed pressure ulcers versus those who do not. As time goes on, the expectation is that every patient will have a daily skin care plan that includes preventive measures without prompting from the skin rounds process. As the culture changes to incorporate these strategies, HAPU rates will stay at zero.

Utilizing a Multifaceted Approach to Improving Nosocomial Pressure Ulcers

Nancy Cann, MSN, RN
Clinical Outcomes Specialist, Nursing Performance Improvement
Nancy.Cann@bmcjax.com

Marsha Miles, MSN, RN, CCRN-CSC
Advanced Practice Partner, Cardiovascular/Thoracic Surgical ICU

Peggy McCartt, MN, CCRN, ARNP
Senior Consultant, Clinical Practice

Teri Billings, RN
Manager, Wound Care Clinic

Baptist Medical Center Downtown

Editor's Pick

INSIGHTS & IDEAS FROM THIS FACILITY

Unit-Based Wound Care Champions and Advanced Practice RNs lead multifaceted pressure ulcer prevention initiative. Emphasis on "hardwiring" admission documentation and risk assessment.

Facility and Unit Summary

Facility	Baptist Medical Center Downtown (BMCD)—Jacksonville, Florida **http://community.e-baptisthealth.com/bmc/downtown/**
Facility setting	Full-service tertiary hospital in downtown Jacksonville with services including cardiology and cardiothoracic surgery; medical, radiation, and surgical oncology; neurosciences; minimally invasive surgery; bloodless medicine and surgery; obstetrics and gynecology; emergency services; orthopedics, and ophthalmology
Teaching status	Nonteaching
Ownership status	Private (Baptist Health)
Community demographics	Service area is primarily southern Duval and northern St. Johns counties, Florida, which includes Jacksonville and St. Augustine, with 80% of the patient population coming from 28 counties. • Race/ethnicity: 56.7% White, 27.7% Black, 7.4% Hispanic, American Indian, 0.9% Asian, and 6.4% other • 1.4 % of service area population over age 65.
Hospital-staffed beds	399
Case mix index (CMI)	1.58
Indicators used	Hospital acquired pressure ulcers
System or unit improved	Three critical care units: Heart 3 South (Coronary Intensive Care), Heart 4 South (Cardiovascular/Thoracic Surgical ICU), and MSICU (Medical Surgical Intensive Care Unit)
Indicator(s) improved	Hospital acquired pressure ulcers
QI documents used	Unit-based progress reports for reporting to staff
NDNQI® participation	Since 2005
Time frame of QI experience	2005–2007
Magnet™ status	Designated December 2007
Governance model	Shared Governance Model

Awards and recognition	• One of *Modern Healthcare's* "100 Best Places to Work in Healthcare" • Accredited as Chest Pain Center by the Society of Chest Pain Centers—2008 • Recipient of the HealthGrades 2008 Distinguished Hospital Award for Clinical Excellence—2008 • Named by Florida Monthly magazine readers as being among their choices for Florida's top healthcare institutions—2008
	• America's Best Hospitals for Digestive Care by *US News & World Report*—2007 • Consumer Choice Award winner for 19 years, based on the National Research Corporation's Health Care Market Guide—2007 • Blue Distinction Center for Cardiac Care by Blue Cross and Blue Shield of Florida—2007

UNIT PROFILES

	Heart 3 South	Heart 4 South	MSICU
Size and type	12 beds; coronary intensive care	24 beds	24 beds
Staff summary	• 68 RNs (60 full-time, 8 part-time) • 15 Acute care technicians (ACPs) • 6 Monitor technicians • 2 Health unit coordinators	• 48 RNs (45 full-time, 3 part-time) • 16 ACPs • 4 Monitor technicians • 2 Health unit coordinators	• 63 RNs (48 full-time, 15 part-time) • 7 ACPs • 2 Health unit coordinators
Staff skill mix	• 52% BSNs • 47% ADNs • 1% diploma • National certifications: 6 • Nurse manager: ARNP	• 59% BSNs • 41% ADNs • National certifications: 4 • Nurse manager: BSN	• 37% BSNs • 56% ADNs • 7% diploma • National certifications: 2 • Nurse manager: BSN
Nurse-patient ratio (NHPPD)	17.49	21.45	16.21
Organizational structure	For all units: Vice President of Patient Care Services, Nursing director, Nurse managers (unit-specific)		

Utilizing a Multifaceted Approach to Improving Nosocomial Pressure Ulcers

Nancy Cann, MSN, RN
Marsha Miles, MSN, RN, CCRN-CSC
Peggy McCartt, MN, CCRN, ARNP
Teri Billings, RN

Baptist Medical Center Downtown

Introductory Summary

Baptist Medical Center Downtown (BMCD) is a 399-bed tertiary care hospital in Jacksonville, Florida, that is part of the only locally governed, faith-based health system in Northeast Florida. A Magnet™ hospital recognized for excellence in patient care, BMCD is the Baptist Health flagship hospital, which includes a total of five hospitals, a home healthcare agency, a network of primary care physicians' offices, and two urgent care centers.

Primarily serving Northeast Florida and Southeast Georgia residents, Baptist Health is accredited by the Joint Commission, which certified the medical center as a Primary Stroke Center in 2007. Baptist includes a number of regional referral centers, including Baptist Heart Hospital, Baptist Cancer Institute, Breast Health Services, Baptist Gamma Knife Center, Jacksonville Orthopaedic Institute, and the Women's Pavilion.

BMCD offers a comprehensive range of medical and surgical services, including but not limited to, cardiology and cardiothoracic surgery; medical, radiation, and surgical oncology; neurosciences; minimally invasive surgery (including the da Vinci® Robotic Surgical System); bloodless medicine and surgery; obstetrics and gynecology; emergency services (including Life Flight, the only air ambulance in Northeast Florida accredited by the Commission for Accreditation of Medical Transport Systems); orthopedics; and ophthalmology. Comprehensive imaging services include two state-of-the-art 64-slice scanners (June 2008) for optimum image quality and patient comfort.

Becoming a member of the National Database of Nursing Quality Indicators® (NDNQI) in the latter part of 2005 was a strategy implemented by Baptist Health during its continuous journey for clinical excellence. Reports for Q2 06 showed patients surveyed within three adult critical care units (Heart 3 South, Heart 4 South, and MSICU) had a median of 18.75% hospital acquired pressure ulcers, with an average of 17.74%.

In a move to improve patient outcomes, the nurse hospitalist role (advanced practice nurses functioning as clinical care managers, who focus on physician documentation and resource utilization) was restructured and evolved into an advanced practice partner (APP) role. The APP brought clinical expertise and resources to the bedside nurse, improving staff nurses' clinical skills and patient outcomes. It was one aspect of the multifaceted approach that was implemented. Other important factors included the work of the wound care nurses, implementation of wound care protocols, identification of wound care unit-based champions, and standardization of wound care products. Lower hospital acquired pressure ulcer rates have been sustained, as evidenced by the adult critical care units following eight quarters (see Table 1).

Clinical Quality Goals

Every year Baptist Health identifies focus areas for clinical improvement. In FY 2007 and 2008, Baptist Health selected hospital acquired pressure ulcers as one of its system clinical focus goals. The first year, FY 2007, the goal was a 25% reduction in hospital acquired pressure ulcers based on a unit's historical rate. The second year, FY 2008, that goal was stretched to achieve a 25% reduction based on the historical rate of the best-performing critical care unit in the health system. The following describes the strategies implemented to achieve these goals and the resulting sustained improvement noted in the statistical data.

Getting Started

Senior administration and nursing leadership support was of critical importance to achieving targeted goals. The first step was the organizational restructuring of the nurse hospitalist and nurse educator roles into unit-based advanced practice partners, which brought much-needed clinical resources to the bedside nurse.

The nurse hospitalist role at Baptist Downtown evolved into a model of care in which there are APPs with similar goals, one of which is to improve patient outcomes. The advanced practice partners are nurses with master's degrees who bring a high level of experience to the clinical units and work directly with staff in partnership with nursing leaders. These APP nurses augmented the model of care and staffing on their assigned units.

As an example, the APPs within the critical care units have embraced the role of patient advocate, expert clinician, and clinical educator while improving compliance with the evidence-based practice standards for pressure ulcer prevention. These objectives were met in a variety of ways. The APPs worked with the nursing staff to ensure that consults, medications, and prevention protocols were addressed in a timely fashion. They also provided critical education to patients and families about their disease process, while fulfilling care coordination and clinical case management-like functions. In addition to working with the wound care team, the APPs facilitated consults to other departments, including dietary and physical therapy. They served as expert clinical resources to the staff nurses—educating them on patients' predisposing factors for possible pressure ulcer risk—while providing and assisting in identifying performance improvement needs and the development of action plans to improve patient outcomes. The APPs also conducted daily rounds with the nursing staff. During rounds, the Braden Scale for Predicting Pressure Sore Risk was reviewed and discussed with the staff to validate the appropriateness of their scoring. This mentoring process of direct care providers has proved to be an essential part of Baptist Health's realization of their clinical goals.

Results

The wound care department assumed responsibility for the NDNQI pressure ulcer point prevalence study during Q2-06. This survey resulted in three critical care units reporting an average of 17.64% patients with hospital acquired pressure ulcers in the same time frame (see Table 1). The NDNQI data were analyzed and an improvement plan developed and implemented. Subsequent to the implementation of the plan, the critical care units have sustained a hospital acquired pressure ulcer prevalence rate below the NDNQI national benchmark, as well as a reduction in the incidence rate.

TABLE 1.
NDNQI Point Prevalence Study Results

Adult Critical Care	Q2–06	Q3–06	Q4–06	Q1–07	Q2–07	Q3–07	Q4–07	1Q08	Avg
Heart 3 South	18.75	7.69	11.11	5.26	0.00	13.33	0.00	0.00	7.02
Heart 4 South	23.08	0.00	0.00	0.00	0.00	0.00	6.67	6.67	4.55
MSICU	11.11	15.79	0.00	5.56	16.67	10.00	10.00	10.00	9.89
Hospital Adult Critical Care Median	*18.75*	*7.69*	*0.00*	*5.26*	*0.00*	*10.00*	*6.67*	*6.67*	*6.88*

Developing Interventions

One of the first areas identified for improvement was the lack of documentation related to admission skin assessment and "present on admission" documentation of pressure ulcers. A random chart audit was conducted for 60 days. Results were reported to the nurse managers and the nursing directors. The enhanced awareness of the need for complete and accurate documentation resulted in a decrease of 5% in the hospital acquired pressure ulcer rates. Having seen how increasing awareness of the importance of documentation could result in such a dramatic improvement, the team began to analyze what other patient-focused interventions might demonstrate an even more positive patient clinical outcome.

Another change in practice was that the wound care team divided the workload for the inpatient wound care nurses and assigned them to particular units. This restructuring by the wound care department allowed the wound care nurses to build relationships with the direct care nurses, unlicensed assistive personnel, physicians, and other consulting departments. The wound care team began rounding on the units daily. "Wound care champions" were identified on the units with high-risk patients. These nurses engaged in peer review of documentation, ensuring that consults to wound care and nutrition were ordered (if appropriate), and educating the staff in best practices (Stoelting et al., 2007). In addition, the Braden scale triggers were adjusted to reflect those patients who might be deemed as high risk or those with comorbidities, so skin care interventions and consults would be implemented sooner (5 Million Lives Campaign, 2008).

In late February 2006, the System Performance Improvement Council, in collaboration with nursing leadership, endorsed a monthly (rather than quarterly) point prevalence study schedule. This decision was supported enthusiastically by hospital administration. The monthly studies were reported to nursing leadership from the unit level to the chief nursing officer and provided timely data on whether the units were reaching benchmarks. Unit nursing leaders shared the data with the direct care nurses at unit council meetings and with the wound care champions. Ultimately, the feedback on progress toward unit goals helped the wound care team provide early interventions to patients, with the intended consequence of improved outcomes.

In addition, the wound care team implemented a monthly educational "Lunch and Learn" program open to all staff, which began the Q1-07. Topics included legal implications of pressure ulcers, nutrition and wound care, and hydrotherapy (Ballard et al., 2007). During these educational opportunities, the team placed reference notebooks on each unit and posted bullet points of information in each staff lounge. The notebooks included pressure ulcer staging information, educational materials including PowerPoint presentations from the Lunch and Learn opportunities, and contact information. These notebooks

FIGURE 1.
PUPP Algorithm

Assessment/Documentation

Documentation of assessment and interventions is essential

- Upon admission to Recovery Bay or unit, every 12 hours, caregiver change or transfer from Recovery Bay to unit bed
- **Confirmed by another RN**
- **Documented on database 2- & 24-hour flow sheet**

***If pressure ulcer develops, initiate Skin Integrity IPOC.**

Braden score 16 or less/
Bedfast patients/ventilator patients

- **Wound care consult ordered**
  - **Braden score**—13 or less
  - **Cardiac surgery patients**—indicate in Special Instructions "s/p heart surgery; call before visit"
  - **Problems with surgical incisions**
  - **Other skin problems**—pressure ulcers, skin tears, perineal dermatitis, tape burns, chemical burns, candida, etc.
- **Shearing**—use **Maxislides** when repositioning pt. Can apply Duoderm to sacral area.
  NOTE: *May apply Benzoin to skin to prevent Duoderm from rolling off skin*
- **Moisture**—Refer to incontinence care
- **Repositioning**
  - Q2 hour using reusable foam wedges. Pillows between knees. NOTE: Avoid placing patient directly on trochanter. **(If skin breakdown on sacrum, DO NOT position on back)**
    - Turning clock in room
    - If patient cannot be turned due to hemodynamic instability, place small pillows under hips and shoulders to relieve pressure
  - Elevate knees before raising HOB. **HOB at 30 degrees**
  - Heels off bed. (**Heel Lift**—order from Cast Tech)
    - May use pillow (temporarily) by placing it lengthwise
- **Nutrition**
  - Dietician consult
  - Daily weights, I&O
- **Early mobility**
  - Passive range of motion unless contraindicated
  - PT/OT consult
  - OOB to chair/ambulation—when hemodynamically stable

Incontinence

- Perineal foam cleanser—**NO** soap and water
- Quickables—**NO** washcloths
- Avoid scrubbing
- Barrier cream—mix ½ Sensicare & ½ Aloe Vesta and apply to skin every 4 hours & PRN
- Dri-Flo pads. **NO** reusable cloth pads
- NO diapers except when ambulating
- Diarrhea/C. difficile—obtain **order** for Flexiseal
- Urinary—condom cath for male patients
- Do not place towels between legs
- Identify fungal infections and obtain order for medications

Skin Tears

- Cleanse with normal saline or wound cleanser
- Apply **Vaseline gauze and Telfa,** then wrap with **Kerlix**

NOTE: DO NOT use Tegaderm.

OOB/Ambulatory

- Pressure-redistribution cushion—**ALL** patients OOB in chair (Order from SPD)
- Shift weight—patients need to shift weight while sitting in chair—every 15 minutes
- Assist to stand—every hour

Pressure-redistribution surface

Use HH4S Screening Tool
to
identify appropriate patients

Device-related Breakdown Prevention:

- Bridge of nose (that is, BiPap)—apply **Duoderm**
- Rim of ear—apply **Duoderm**

FIGURE 2.

Screening Tool for Assessing Need for Specialty Mattress

HH4S Screening Tool for Specialty Bed/Mattress

All orders for specialty beds/mattresses must be approved by APP, ANM, NM or Wound Care

DATES:									
If patient has one of the following, an order should be placed for one of the beds listed below:									
Nonblanchable redness									
• Reposition pt. and recheck in 30 minutes. (If no change and pt. at high risk for shearing)									
Pressure ulcer present (stage 2 or higher, DTI)									
If 3 or more of the following criteria are present, an order should be placed for one of the beds listed below:									
Mechanical ventilation more than 24 hrs. *No possibility of extubation within the next 24 hrs.									
IABP									
Infusions of vasopressors									
Neuromuscular blockade									
3 or more comorbidities— (Hx CVA, DM, ecchymosis, renal insufficiency/ failure, heart failure, respiratory disease, PVD)									
Hospitalized with bedrest for more than 24 hours prior to surgery									
Age greater than 60									
More than 4 hours on OR table									

Types of beds mattresses available:

- **Envision E-700 low air loss mattress (less than 300 lbs)—fits Total Care bed**
- **Total Care Bariatric with air (300 lbs or greater)**
- **Tri-Flex—for patients 6'3 and taller (must order the whole bed)**

Patient Label

FIGURE 3.

Baptist Health Wound Care Web Site

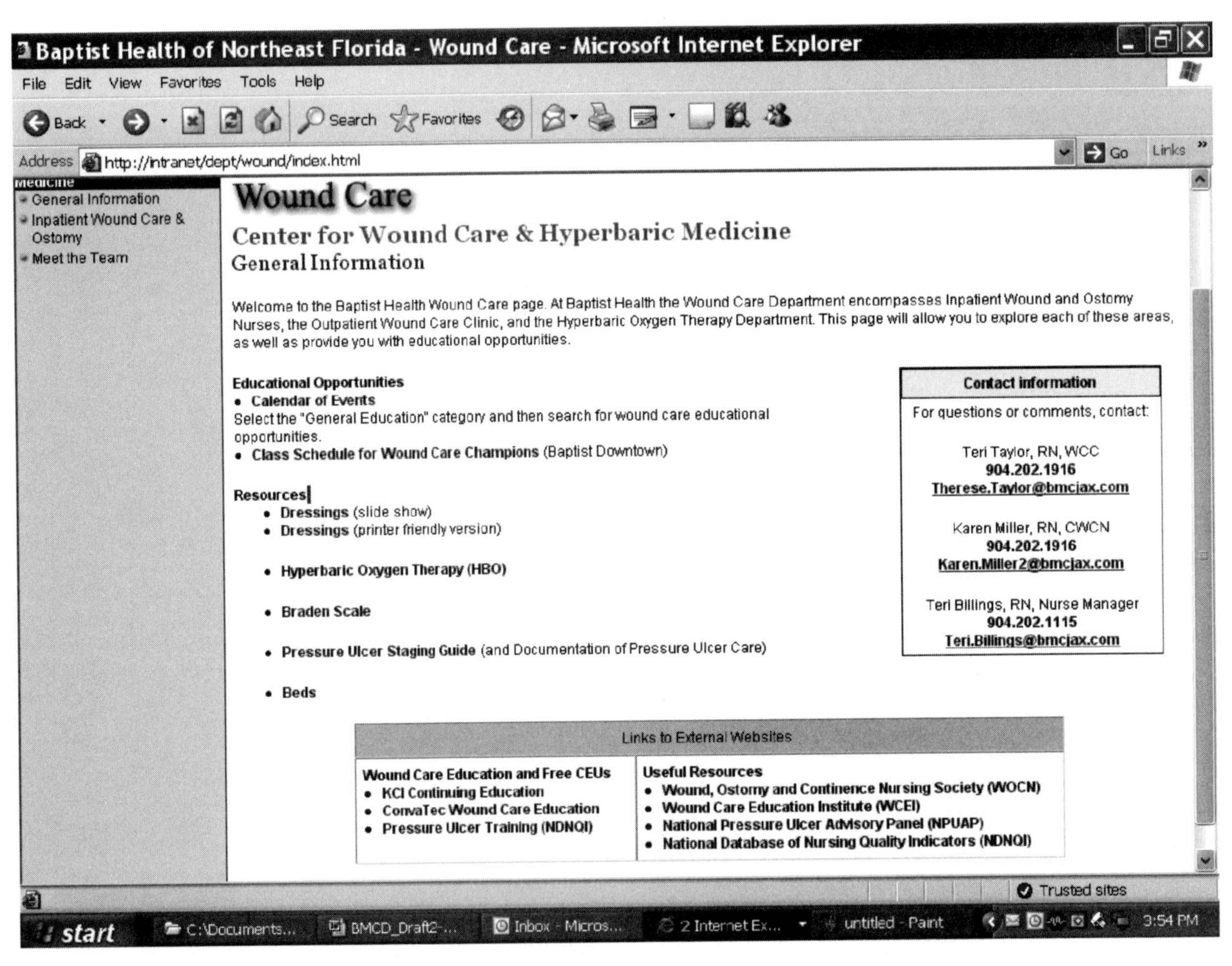

have now been updated with the screening tool for specialty mattresses/beds and the wound care algorithm (Keast et al., 2007). The wound care team, in conjunction with an outside consultant, implemented the use of foam wedges as a pilot in the critical care units with much success. Research has shown effective turning reduces pressure on the bony prominences, which is considered best practice in the prevention of pressure ulcers. Foam wedges are utilized to maintain proper positioning (Catania et al., 2007)

Next Steps: Hardwiring the Process

The advanced practice partners for Heart 3 South (Coronary Intensive Care), Heart 4 South (Cardiovascular/Thoracic Surgical ICU), and MSICU (Medical Surgical Intensive Care Unit) were responsible for identifying trends in patient care and improving outcomes. The APPs collaborated with the wound care team, which resulted in the development of additional pressure ulcer initiatives. These included a literature review related to risk factors for pressure ulcer development, especially in critical care and cardiac surgery patients, and prevention techniques.

Based on the literature review, a unit-based Pressure Ulcer Prevention Protocol (PUPP) with a screening tool for specialty bed/pressure redistribution mattresses for postoperative cardiovascular surgery patients was developed (Feuchtinger, Halfens, & Dassen, 2005; Frankel, Sperry, & Kaplan, 2007). The APPs for the critical care units developed a PUPP algorithm (see Figure 1) to assist the bedside nurse in assessing the need for a specialty mattress (see Figure 2).

- The PUPP algorithm incorporates the six key steps identified by the Institute of Healthcare Improvement's 5 Million Lives Campaign (2008) to prevent pressure ulcers. These steps include pressure ulcer admission assessment, daily reassessment, daily skin inspection, moisture management, nutrition and hydration optimization, and minimization of pressure to the skin. The algorithm provides the bedside nurse with potential skin breakdown interventions.
- Using a daily risk assessment tool as shown here allows the provider to implement strategies based on the patient's daily reassessment. An example might be that after several days in the hospital, a patient's ability to get out of bed has been altered by an intervention, such as hip replacement surgery. This quick guide enables the bedside nurse to quickly identify the patient's status change and implement the appropriate skin breakdown prevention intervention.

Research has shown that patients with three or more comorbidities, older than 60, and in the operating room for more than 4 hours are at increased risk for skin breakdown. The cardiovascular APP developed a screening tool for a specialty bed/mattress based on this evidence and the knowledge of admitted patients to her unit. The tool provides the bedside nurse information related to type of bed/mattress that should be ordered based on the type of bed the patient is presently occupying. The assessment/screening tool eliminated confusion over the type of bed/mattress that needed to be ordered.

FIGURE 4.
Turn/Position Clock

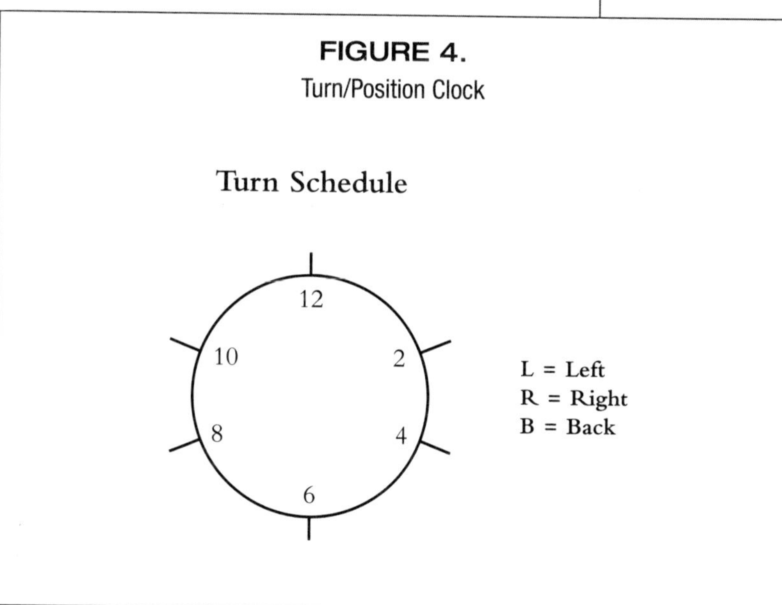

Staff education was provided through nursing and ancillary staff in-services, journal clubs, and weekly interdisciplinary and daily APP rounds (Wolverton et al., 2004) A web site was created for the wound care department, enhancing staff access to information related to pressure ulcers (see Figure 3).

To further hardwire the importance of documentation of the patient's skin at admission, a contest was conducted to increase staff completion of the initial Braden skin breakdown assessment scale. If documentation was completed at admission and the unit sustained the documentation for 30 days in a row, each shift was given a meal catered by a local restaurant. Other process changes to improve staff assessment and interventions included placement of a paper turning/positioning clock (see Figure 4) in patients' rooms as a reminder to staff to turn patients on every even hour.

Other interventions included a wound care consult for all cardiac surgery patients upon admission from the cardiovascular operating room. The wound ostomy continence (WOC) nurse contacts the direct care nurse on post-op day 1. Most of these patients are ambulatory and the Braden score is greater than 16. But if the patient is still on a ventilator, with limited ability for independent movement, the WOC nurse assesses the patient for possible further skin care interventions.

Education was conducted, not just for the bedside nurse but also for those in nursing leadership positions. Four times a year, Baptist Health nursing leadership conducts a Nursing Leadership Academy (NLA). NLA is a forum for all nurse leaders, including nurse directors, nurse managers, assistant nurse managers, educators, performance improvement coordinators, and others to review best practices to allow those in key leadership positions to support the work of the nurse at the bedside. Baptist Health Clinical Quality Goals, which included hospital acquired pressure ulcers, was the topic for the fall 2007 Nursing Leadership Academy. Prior to attending the 4-hour program, attendees completed the NDNQI Pressure Ulcer Training Module. Certificates of successful completion were required and entered into the nursing leaders' profile for educational tracking purposes. The speaker conducted a literature review for best practices that were included in the presentation. Evidence-based best practices were presented with a "call to action" for nursing management. The Risk Management and Patient Safety Division presented Patient Safety Grand Rounds on pressure ulcers. The 1-hour program presented by Baptist Health risk managers was offered to all staff throughout Baptist Health via videoconferencing, further emphasizing the importance of documentation and of implementing prevention protocols when patients are identified as at risk. These multifaceted educational approaches provided additional forums to get the word out about the importance of pressure ulcer prevention and the importance related to patient care.

The Systemwide Performance Improvement Council created a "Quality Rounds" audit form to monitor the progress of the clinical system goals. This form was completed by the nurse manager or designee on each nursing unit. Five charts per week were audited for documentation of skin assessment. If a patient was identified as at risk for skin breakdown based on the Braden scale, an evaluation was done on whether the appropriate interventions had been implemented and documented. These included a turning schedule, specialty bed or pressure redistribution mattress, heels-off bed, consult to wound care nurse, and nutrition and physical therapy consults, if indicated.

The data were presented and made available to the nurse managers, and the hospital and system-level PI councils. The information was shared with the direct care nurses in staff meetings and was included on the unit progress reports. NDNQI data were used in the improvement plan as external benchmarks and also included on the unit progress reports.

Where Baptist Health Is Today

Baptist Health continues to use NDNQI reports for benchmarking. The new reports allow benchmarking not only against like units in same-size hospitals but also against Magnet-designated facilities. Baptist Health strives to achieve outcomes in the top quartile.

Today, Baptist Health has 44 trained "Wound Care Champions" hospitalwide. These wound care champions are staff nurses who have volunteered to "step it up and step it out" in achieving clinical excellence. They serve as a resource for their peers and assist with the monthly point prevalence study. They also are responsible for the white status boards, which have been placed on all the units, displaying the number of days free of hospital acquired pressure ulcers.

The Advanced Practice Council, which comprises the APPs and clinical effectiveness, performance improvement, and clinical outcomes specialists, developed a multidisciplinary matrix to focus on the incidence of hospital acquired pressure ulcers. Wound care products and a supply list were developed and are available on all units. This has provided direct care nurses easy access to the supplies needed to maintain skin integrity and to care for patients at risk for and with skin breakdown.

Conclusion and Implications

The NDNQI quarterly reports reflect a sense of accomplishment for the bedside nurses and interdisciplinary team that has resulted in better patient outcomes. Pressure ulcer initiatives have been implemented not only hospitalwide but across the health system. Consequences of better patient outcomes, as reflected by the reduction in hospital acquired pressure ulcers, mean reduced costs and improved revenue. This is even more important in light of the Centers for Medicare and Medicaid Services (CMS) payment schedule for hospital acquired conditions. Better patient outcomes can affect not only patient satisfaction scores but RN satisfaction scores, as nurses can see evidence of their quality of care through internal dashboards and progress reports. The APP role was the driving force in achieving a reduction in hospital acquired pressure ulcers in the three critical care units profiled. Their expertise has been invaluable to the staff and interdisciplinary team in providing leadership in meeting quality goals as well as professional development of staff (Ayello & Lyder, 2008).

References

Ayello, E. A., & Lyder, C. H. (2008). A new era of pressure ulcer accountability in acute care. *Advances in Skin and Wound Care, 21*(3), 134–140.

Ballard, N., McCombs, A., DeBoor, S., Strachan, J., Johnson, M., Smith, M. J., et al. (2007). How our ICU decreased the rate of hospital-acquired pressure ulcers. *Journal of Nursing Care Quality, 23*(1), 92–96.

Catania, K., Huang, C., James, P., Ohr, M., Madison, M., & Moran, M. (2007). PUPPI: The pressure ulcer prevention protocol interventions. *American Journal of Nursing, 107*(4), 44–52.

Feuchtinger, J., Halfens, R. J. G., & Dassen, T. (2005). Pressure ulcer risk factors in cardiac surgery: A review of the research literature. Heart and Lung, 34, 375–385.

Frankel, H., Sperry, J., & Kaplan, L. (2007). Risk factors for pressure ulcer development in a best practice surgical intensive care unit. *The American Surgeon, 73*, 1215–1217.

5 Million Lives Campaign. (2008). *Getting started kit: Prevent pressure ulcers how-to guide.* Cambridge, MA: Institute for Healthcare Improvement. Retrieved January 9, 2009, from http://www.ihi.org/nr/rdonlyres/5ababb51-93b3-4d88-ae19-be88b7d96858/0/pressureulcerhowtoguide.doc

Keast, D. H., Parslow, N., Houghton, P. E., Norton, L., & Fraser, C. (2007). Best practice recommendations for the prevention and treatment of pressure ulcers: Update 2006. *Advances in Skin and Wound Care, 20*(8), 447–462.

Stoelting, J., McKenna, L., Taggart, E., Mottar, R., Jeffers, B. R., & Wendler, M. C. (2007). Prevention of nosocomial pressure ulcers. *Journal of Wound Ostomy Continence Nursing, 34*(4), 382–388.

Wolverton, C. L., Hobbs, L. A., Beeson, T., Benjamin, M., Campbell, K., Forbes, C., et al. (2004). Nosocomial pressure ulcer rates in critical care: Performance improvement project. *Journal of Nursing Care Quality, 20*(1), 56–62.

Patient Falls

Defined:

A patient fall is an unplanned descent to the floor (or extension of the floor, e.g., trash can or other equipment) with or without injury to the patient, and occurs on an eligible reporting nursing unit. All types of falls are to be included whether they result from physiological reasons (fainting) or environmental reasons (slippery floor). Include assisted falls, such as when a staff member attempts to minimize the impact of the fall.

Exclude falls by:

- Visitors
- Students
- Staff members
- Patients on units not eligible for reporting
- Patients from eligible reporting unit; however, patient was not on the unit at time of the fall (e.g., patient falls in radiology department)

Injury Falls:

Injury level classified as None, Minor, Moderate, Major, or Death.

Formula:

- Total Falls: (Number of Patient Falls X 1000)/Total Number of Patient Days
- Injury Falls: (Number of Patient Injury Falls X 1000)/Total Number of Patient Days

Achieving Sustained Reduction in Patient Falls

Grace Anderson, RN, MS, CCRN
Clinical Director, Heart & Vascular Institute
Grace.Anderson@memorialhermann.org

Tammy Campos, RN, MSN
Clinical Director, MICU, MIMU, TSICU, Rapid Response Team, Code Team, SWAT

Virginia Earley, RN, MSN, CMSRN
Clinical Director, Medicine Services

Dawn Johantges, RN, BSN, CCRN
Clinical Director, Trauma Services

Cathy L. Johnson, RN, BSN
Clinical Manager, CVIMU

Erica O'Connor, MPH
Project Manager
Nursing Administration

The Memorial Hermann Healthcare System,
Texas Medical Center

Editor's Pick

INSIGHTS & IDEAS FROM THIS FACILITY

Staff education on the importance of risk assessment and a range of prevention strategies that can be tailored to each patient's circumstance lead to reduction in fall rates.

Facility and Unit Summary

Facility	Memorial Hermann—Texas Medical Center (MH-TMC), Houston, TX **www.memorialhermann.org/locations/texasmedicalcenter**
Facility setting	MH-TMC serves the greater Houston area with strengths in heart, neuroscience, orthopedics, women's health care, general surgery, and organ transplantation. A certified Level I trauma center, providing 24-hour emergency and trauma care to more than 40,000 patients a year, with air ambulance service, provides emergency rescue and air transport services to a multicounty area.
Teaching status	Primary teaching hospital for the University of Texas Medical School at Houston
Ownership status	Not-for-profit
Community demographics	Primary service area is Brazoria, Fort Bend, Harris, Liberty and Montgomery counties of South Texas. Within the primary service area the largest ethnic groups are Caucasian (37.5%), Hispanic (36.3%), and Black/African American (18.1%), with an estimated overall population of over 4 million people. Approximately 7.4% of service area population over age 65.
Hospital-staffed beds	594 adult patient beds
Case mix index (CMI)	2.16
Indicators used	Patient fall rates
System or unit improved	Three units improved (Critical Care Medical ICU (MICU), Cardiovascular Intermediate Care Unit (CVIMU), and 6 East Jones—Ortho-Trauma (Surgical)
Indicator improved	Patient fall rates
QI documents used	NDNQI benchmark fall rates
NDNQI® participation	Since January 2003
Magnet™ status	Submitting application in 2009
Governance model	Shared Governance (formal, council-based)

Awards and recognition	• Pathway to Excellence designation from American Nurses Credentialing Center—2008 • US News & World Report's "America's Best Hospitals"—2007 • Center ranked 39th in Urology—2007 • Thomson 100 Top Hospitals Performance Improvement Leader—2007 • Thomson 100 Top Hospitals: Cardiovascular Benchmarks for Success study (Heart and Vascular Institute)—2007 • VHA Leadership Awards—for clinical excellence and for community benefit—2007 • Texas Health Care Quality Improvement Award of Excellence—2007

UNIT PROFILE

	MICU (Medical)	CVIMU (Surgical)	6 EAST JONES—ORTHO-TRAUMA (Surgical)
Size and type	16-bed medical intensive care unit	17-bed cardiovascular surgery intermediate care unit with physiologic monitoring	33-bed orthopedic and trauma floor unit
Staff summary (FTEs)			
Licensed vocational nurses	0.9	0.9	4.5
Registered nurses	32.4	19.4	42
Unit clerks	2.7	2.3	6.3
Patient care assistants	4.5	5.5	17.2
Clinical manager	1.0	1.0	1.0
Staff skill mix			
% RNs	70%	75%	60%
% LVNs	5%	5%	10%
% Certified	15% CCRN	—	2% TNCC
% ADNs	15%	53%	30%
% BSN	75%	47%	60%
% MSN	5%	0%	0%
Nurse-patient ratios			
RN–patient	1:1 to 1:3	1:4	1:5 to 1:6

Organizational structure	Chief Patient Care Officer, Associate Patient Care Officer, Nursing director, Nursing managers

Achieving Sustained Reduction in Patient Falls

Grace Anderson, RN, MS, CCRN
Tammy Campus, RN, MSN
Virginia Earley, RN, MSN, CMSRN
Dawn Johantges, RN, BSN, CCRN
Cathy L. Johnson, RN, BSN
Erica O'Connor, MPH

The Memorial Hermann Healthcare System, Texas Medical Center

Introductory Summary

One of the largest healthcare systems in the greater Houston/Galveston metropolitan area of South Texas, the Memorial Hermann Healthcare System (MHHS) consists of 14 community hospitals, a substance abuse center, and dozens of specialty and outpatient centers. As the MHHS presence in the Texas Medical Center, the MH-TMC campus consists of 594 adult patient beds and is the primary teaching hospital for the University of Texas Medical School at Houston. As one of only two certified Level I trauma centers in the greater Houston area, the hospital provides 24-hour emergency and trauma care to more than 40,000 patients a year. Memorial Hermann Life Flight® air ambulance service operates a fleet of six helicopters, providing emergency rescue and air transport services to a multicounty area. For over 100 years, MHHS has provided health services to residents of Houston and surrounding communities. As an indicator of the commitment to quality improvement held by MHHS, in August 2007 the MH-TMC facility was named to the list of Thomson 100 Top Hospitals: Performance Improvement Leaders and is the only facility in Houston to hold a place on that list. Also in 2007, MH-TMC received two Voluntary Hospitals of America (VHA) Leadership Awards, for clinical excellence and for community benefit, as well as the Texas Health Care Quality Improvement Award of Excellence.

Quality improvement has been a driving force for MH-TMC for several years. It is a continuous process and can be found in initiatives that span all levels of the campus. New construction, electronic medical records, and direct patient care are all centered on providing high quality and creating excellent patient outcomes. At MH-TMC, quality outcomes are not just talked about, but are lived, breathed, and practiced.

The Starting Point

In the fall of 2004, the Joint Commission released patient safety goals for hospitals for 2005. Included on this list for the first time was Goal 9: Reduce the risk of patient harm resulting from falls (JCAHO, 2004). Discussion in the Quality and Safety Excellence Council, a subset of the Clinical Practice Steering Council, called for the formation of a subcommittee to address patient falls in early 2005. To ensure a multidisciplinary approach to fall prevention, membership on this committee included representatives from clinical nursing staff, nursing education, physical therapy, pharmacy, facilities management, performance improvement, and

TABLE 1.
Falls per 1,000 Patient Days
MH-TMC and NDNQI Rates—Hospitals with 500+ Staffed Beds
Q3-04 and Q4-04
Adult Unit Types

	Critical Care Medical ICU (MICU)	Step-Down Cardiovascular Intermediate Care (CVIM)	Surgical Ortho-Trauma (6EJ)
MH-TMC	0.98	n.d.	1.77
NDNQI	1.23	3.06	2.66

n.d. = no data.

nursing management. The fall reduction committee was charged with reviewing historical fall data for the facility and comparing it with national data, reviewing current literature, reviewing current facility practice, and developing best practice recommendations for implementation.

The fall reduction committee had compared fall rates of each of the nursing units to NDNQI benchmarks for the unit type. To gain further insight into patient population risk, they scrutinized the data more closely for specific unit differences in patient acuity. To capture data across the continuum of care, units were divided by acuity into three categories:

- Critical care—included all intensive care units
- Intermediate care—included all intermediate and step-down units
- General acute care—included all general floor level of care units

By using these three categories, different types of patient fall risks were identified readily in different patient populations. Data examined included all aspects of the fall, including patient location, age, gender, diagnosis, and activity at the time of the fall. Additional considerations were previous history of falling, medications during hospitalization, witnessed or unwitnessed fall, level of consciousness prior to and at the time of the fall, lighting of surroundings, and any impairment in mobility.

Sample data from one representative unit in each of the acuity categories gave the following data for fall rates in the last 6 months of 2004 (see Table 1).

Although the data indicated fall rates in this sample at MH-TMC to be at or below NDNQI averages, it was felt that a reduction in fall rates could be achieved and sustained with a hospitalwide focus to identify at-risk patients and proactively implement interventions to prevent falls.

The Evidence Base

A review of the literature proved to be of minimal assistance, as many studies were not generalizable to different patient populations. One significant finding identified in the literature was the consistent use of a valid tool for fall risk assessment. Research published in the *International Journal of Nursing Practice* (McFarlane-Kolb, 2004) partially validated the use of the Morse Fall Scale as a tool that was easily adaptable and transferable for use in detecting fall risk in different patient populations. Because the information developed via literature review failed to provide solid recommendations on best practice, it was decided to examine successful practices in use at regional facilities.

An examination of current practice to prevent patient falls at MH-TMC included the use of a fall assessment form that was developed internally by the nursing management team and Nursing Education Department. However, there was no clear-cut standard practice for fall prevention and interventions done on an individual unit basis.

The Intervention Plan

The fall reduction committee returned to the Quality and Safety Excellence Council with the following recommendations for immediate implementation.

First, the Morse Fall Scale assessment should be completed on admission and every 24 hours.

Second, when patients are identified to be at risk for a fall, nursing staff has an assortment of interventions to select from to tailor the intervention plan to the individual needs of the specific patient. Those interventions include the following:

- Falling star decal placed on door of patient's room for patients with a Morse score of > 25
- Two falling star decals placed on door of patient's room for patients who have experienced a fall during their current hospital stay (to heighten awareness)
- Yellow patient armband to identify fall risk patients
- Placement of patients at risk of falling in proximity to each other for frequent observation
- Placement of patients at risk of falling near nursing station in centralized units
- Involvement of family as caregivers, and encouraged family presence 24 hours/day
- Use of one-on-one sitters as deemed necessary
- Hourly rounding, offering frequent hydration and scheduled bathroom assistance
- Adequate lighting in room and bathroom
- Fall risk status discussed in shift change report and team shift huddles every 12 hours

In conjunction with these recommendations, the fall reduction committee also requested that an intense staff education program be developed to ensure that the Morse assessment is completed in a timely fashion and accurately and that the appropriate interventions are implemented.

TABLE 2.
Falls per 1,000 Patient Days, for Selected MH-TMC Units, 2004–2007

	Q3/Q4-04	2005	2006	2007
Critical Care MICU	0.98	1.42	1.51	0.49
Step-Down, CVIMU	n.d.	1.93	3.47	1.79
Surgical, Ortho-Trauma (6 East Jones)	1.77	3.12	2.59	1.25

The education task was the responsibility of the Nursing Education Department for development and rollout to nursing units. As a means to give up-to-date feedback to staff regarding the effectiveness of interventions, a monthly nursing report card was posted on the hospital shared computer drive so staff could compare units in the hospital to NDNQI data.

The Outcomes

In 2007, all three units demonstrated a downward trend after aggressive screening and implementation of the fall prevention initiative commenced (see Table 2).

While trends weren't always in the same direction from year to year, between the last half of 2004 and 2007, fall rates had been reduced by half in MICU and by 29% in the surgical unit 6 East Jones (see Figure 1). Fall rates varied widely from year to year on the CVIMU, but 2007 rates were 8% lower than 2005. In 2007, all three units showed patient fall rates below their particular NDNQI comparison group as well as below the 2004 rates, just before the patient fall reduction committee was created.

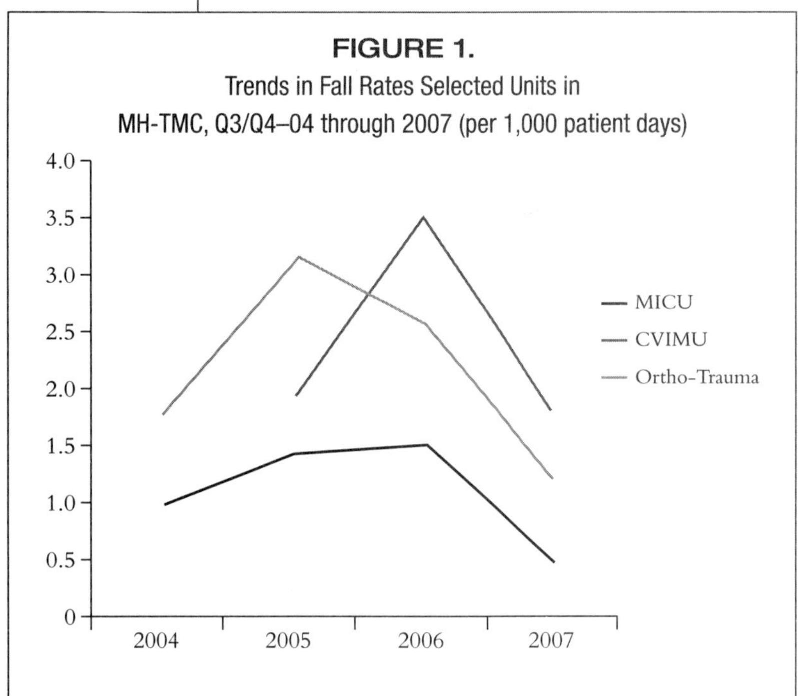

FIGURE 1.
Trends in Fall Rates Selected Units in
MH-TMC, Q3/Q4–04 through 2007 (per 1,000 patient days)

The benefit from a reduction in fall rates for patients at MH-TMC is clear. Decreased fall rates equate to lower risk of injury to patients. Previous studies have found that injuries occurred to patients in 30% of falls, and severe injuries in 4% to 6% of patient falls (Morse, 2002; Schwendimann, Buhler, De Geest, & Milisen, 2006). Injuries from falls resulted in an increased length of stay (LOS) of 12.3 days, or 61%. According to Titler et al. (2005), a safety reduction program saves $432 per fall prevented. Financial costs related to possible litigation related to a fall or any postdischarge cost could be extremely significant and vary by case. A hospital could be forced to pay a settlement if a patient or the patient's family sued the hospital and won on grounds of negligence related to a fall. Using the adjusted Bates estimates for calculation, the cost of each patient fall, regardless of injury, would be $612/per patient fall in 2007 dollars.[1] Given this information, cost avoidance may be calculated for the reduction of patient falls at MH-TMC. For the baseline year of 2004, the three units under review had a total of 34 patient falls, with an associated cost of $20,793. In 2005, these same units had 47 total falls, with an estimated cost of $28,742. In 2007, there were 25 falls, with an associated cost of $15,289. Although these figures might appear small, they are based on falls from three patient care units, or 157 patient beds, in a hospital with 594 patient beds.

The Continuous Process

While proud of these results, the team knew that quality improvement was a journey and not a destination, so continuous quality improvement was pursued. The Patient Fall Reduction Program Committee meets biweekly and reviews all incidents of falling, looking for trends and opportunities for improvement. The data are analyzed on a monthly basis and presented to the overall facility quality improvement council. Recommendations are then communicated to the clinical director, manager, and nursing staff of each unit that has an upward trend in fall data. Those units identified with upward trends will initiate the "fall bundle" to decrease their rates the next month.

During the committee's annual review of 2007 data it was determined that the majority of falls at MH-TMC occurred on the inpatient rehabilitation unit. The fall risk for patients with intrinsic risk factors can be predicted most accurately by the use of a risk assessment tool (Rutledge & Matteucci, 2008). Thus, patients housed on an inpatient rehabilitation unit are not only at increased intrinsic risk, but could also benefit from the implementation of prevention protocols if identified as at risk through the use of the Morse Fall Scale. As a result, the most recent recommendations from the fall reduction committee to be used housewide included:

1. Bates et al. (1995) estimated additional costs to be $4,233 per patient who fell. That study was based on data collected from January 1987 through March 1991. Using 1989 as the midpoint of that period, the authors have adjusted his results to 2007 dollars, using the ratio of the consumer price index for 1989 and 2007.

- Morse Fall Scale reevaluation every 12 hours (increased from every 24 hours)
- "High risk for fall" medication alerts
- Bowel and bladder protocol for assistance getting to and from the bathroom
- Bed exit alarms
- Low Boy beds for high-risk patients
- Busy vests to occupy patients as a deterrent to exiting the bed
- Night lights for high-risk patients
- Florescent floor tape to identify the pathway to the bathroom
- Double nonskid socks (beige) for all patients at risk for falls
- Double nonskid socks (red) for all patients who have experienced a fall during their hospital stay, to heighten staff and family awareness
- Implementation of a "fall bundle" for all patients with a Morse score greater than 25 and a separate bundle for patients with a Morse score greater than 50

Lessons Learned

The past 3 years have demonstrated that there is no single change in patient care that is successful in preventing patient falls. Each occasion of a fall is as different as the patient and circumstances involved. Each patient must be assessed and frequently reassessed to identify circumstances that place the patient at risk and to select the best interventions to prevent falls.

Conclusions and Implications

The most well-designed interventions for fall prevention are ineffective if they are not selected and implemented appropriately. At MH-TMC, three factors were key to its success: an engaged workforce, comparative data, and continuous feedback. At the heart of the fall reduction program is an engaged workforce. The bedside nurse must recognize that he or she is the first line of defense for patients against a fall injury. When the nurse is vigilant in assessment and intervention, the risks to the patient are decreased. Comparative data provided the impetus for change. While the use of unit-to-unit comparisons is motivating, the inclusion of national benchmarking can be even more so.

Of special interest is the fact that during this process improvement, a reduction goal was never identified to staff. Data for all units were published with comparison to NDNQI unit-type data. The comparisons themselves motivated the staff to do better. A final factor is ongoing feedback. Fall data are frequently discussed at staff meetings, nurse council meetings, and performance improvement councils, and opportunities are explored and shared throughout the facility. In response, the staff took the responsibility for fall reduction at the bedside and achieved laudable results.

References

Bates, D., Pruess, K., Souney, P., & Platt, R. (1995). Serious falls in hospitalized patients: Correlates and resource utilization. *American Journal of Medicine, 99*, 137–143.

The Joint Commission. (2004). 2005 Hospital National Patient Safety Goals. Retrieved January 9, 2009, from http://www.jointcommission.org/PatientSafety/NationalPatientSafetyGoals/05_hap_npsgs.htm

McFarlane-Kolb, H. (2004). Falls risk assessment, multitargeted interventions and the impact on hospital falls. *International Journal of Nursing Practice, 10*(5), 199–206.

Morse, J. (2002). Enhancing the safety of hospitalization by reducing patient falls. *American Journal of Infection Control, 30*(6), 376–380.

Rutledge, D., & Matteucci, R. (2008). Fall prevention in hospitalized patients. In D. Pravikoff (Ed.) (pp. 2p). Glendale, CA: Cinahl Information Systems.

Schwendimann, R., Buhler, H., De Geest, S., & Milisen, K. (2006). Falls and consequent injuries in hospitalized patients: Effects of an interdisciplinary falls prevention program. *BMC Health Services Research, 6*, 69.

Titler, M., Dochterman, J., Picone, D. M., Everett, L., Xie, X., Kanak, M., & Fei, Q. (2005). Cost of hospital care for the elderly at risk of falling. *Nursing Economics, 23*(6), 290–306.

Background Resources

Burritt, J., et al. (2007). Achieving quality and fiscal outcomes in patient care: The Clinical Mentor Care Delivery model. *Journal of Nursing Administration, 37*(12), 558–563.

Iglesias, C. P., Manca, A., & Torgerson, D. (2008). The health-related quality of life and cost implications of falls in elderly women. *Osteoporosis International* (October).

Stevens, J. A., et al. (2006). The costs of fatal and non-fatal falls among older adults. *Injury Prevention, 12*, 290–295. (doi:10.1136/ip.2005.011015)

Watts, J. et al. (2008). Cost effectiveness of preventing falls and improving mobility in people with Parkinson disease: A protocol of an economic evaluation alongside a clinical trial. *BMC Geriatrics, 8*, 23. (doi: 10.1186/1471-2318-8-23)

Fall Reduction Strategies: Using a Rapid Cycle FOCUS-PDSA Process to Reduce Patient Falls

Carol Gouty, RN, MSN, PhD, CAN-BC
Director of Nursing Professional Practice
Carol_A_Gouty@rsh.net

Judi Bonomi, RN, MS, MSN, OCN
Director, Inpatient Nursing, CCC/MSU/ONP

Dabney Messer-Rehak, PT, MS, CHE
Administrative Director, Physical Medicine and Rehabilitation Center

Robin Garcia
Administrative Assistant, Nursing Professional Practice

Rush-Copley Medical Center

Editor's Pick

INSIGHTS & IDEAS FROM THIS FACILITY

Staff nurses led the culture change from "falls happen" to "patient falls will not occur in our hospital." Rapid cycle quality improvement process identified a wide variety of practice changes needed to reduce falls.

Facility and Unit Summary

Facility	Rush-Copley Medical Center (RCMC)—Aurora, Illinois **www.rushcopley.com**
Facility setting	A full-service RCMC features the only Level III neonatal intensive care unit in Kane County performing 4,000 births/year. An extensive emergency facility handles over 60,000 patients/year.
Teaching status	Family practice residency program, the only one in the greater Fox Valley area
Ownership status	Tax exempt, not-for-profit
Community demographics	Suburban community located in Aurora, 35 miles west of Chicago; primary service area: Kane County (pop. 323,877); secondary service area: Kendall County (pop 176,158 people). • Largest race/ethnic groups served in the total service area: Caucasian (76%), Hispanic (23%), African American (7%) • Population of total service area considered to be low-income: 10–13; underserved population in primary service area: 36% • Approximately 8.4% of primary service area and 7.3% of secondary over age 65
Hospital-staffed beds	183 beds
Case mix index (CMI)	Medicare, 1.55; overall, 1.04
Indicators used	Falls, Pressure Ulcers and Restraints, Nursing Hours, Certification and Education, RN Satisfaction
System or unit improved	Falls in the combined medical/surgical units of the Cancer Care Center (CCC), Medical/Surgical Pediatrics (MSP; redesignated Ortho/Neuro Peds [ORP] in January 2008), and Inpatient Rehabilitation (Physical Rehabilitation Center; [PHC])
Indicator improved	Total fall rate for CY 2007 improved in all three units; 616 days without a patient fall resulting in a major injury, as of November 12, 2008
QI documents used	NDNQI and departmental scorecards
NDNQI® participation	Since July 2002

Time frame of QI experience	September 2006 through December 2007
Magnet™ status	Activities under way with goal to achieve designation by 2011
Governance model	Partnership Model (a shared governance structure)
Awards and recognition	• Recognized for fourth consecutive year in "100 Most Wired Hospitals and Health Systems" by Hospitals and Health Networks—2007 • JD Power and Associates recognition as a "Distinguished Provider of an Outstanding Patient Experience" (the only Illinois hospital to have received this distinction 2 years in a row)—2006, 2007

UNIT PROFILE

Staff summary	All licensed, professional registered nurses (RNs), with 55% of the RNs holding a Bachelor of Science or higher; RNs on each unit provide patient care with the support of clinical associates (CAs)

	CCC (Cancer Care Center)	MSP (Med/Surg Peds)	PHC (Inpatient Rehabilitation)
Size and type	24 beds; oncology and medical/surgical overflow unit	36 beds; orthopedic and general medical/surgical unit, with 6 beds for pediatric patients	12 beds; inpatient rehabilitation unit
Staff skill mix	70% RNs	70% RNs	60% RNs
Nurse-patient ratio (NHPPD)	10.38 • 1 RN: 4 to 5 patients • 1 CA: 7 to 8 patients	10.01 • 1 RN: 6 patients • 1 CA: 6 patients	9.05
Organizational structure	Chief nursing officer, Director, Nurse manager; each unit has a nurse manager who has 30 to 110 direct reports		

Fall Reduction Strategies: Using a Rapid Cycle FOCUS-PDSA Process to Reduce Patient Falls

Carol Gouty, RN, MSN, PhD, CAN-BC
Judi Bonomi, RN, MS, MSN, OCN
Dabney Messer-Rehak, PT, MS, CHE
Robin Garcia

Rush-Copley Medical Center

Introductory Summary

Rush-Copley Medical Center (RCMC) is a 183-bed facility situated on a 100-acre campus in Aurora, the second largest city in Illinois. Located 35 miles west of Chicago, RCMC serves a diverse population of 500,035 people—323,877 people in the primary service area and 176,158 people in the secondary service area. The three largest ethnic groups served in the total service area are Caucasian (76%), Hispanic (23%), and African American (7%). Primary service lines include cardiology, oncology, orthopedics, neuroscience, and women's health. Of the area's population, 10% to 13% are considered low income, and 36% of the residents in the primary service area are considered to be underserved. RCMC's mission is to provide advanced medicine with quality outcomes and extraordinary nursing care. Quality outcomes and extraordinary care result in part from RCMC's commitment to providing a safe patient care environment, which includes a patient experience free of falls.

Background

RCMC has participated in NDNQI since July 2002 to compare its performance with facilities recognized for nursing excellence. Goals were established for nursing-sensitive indicators using a benchmark of performance reported through the NDNQI database.

In September 2006, staff and leadership recognized that progress in reducing falls—from a high of 10–18 falls per month in the two inpatient medical/surgical (med/surg) units and the Inpatient Rehabilitation unit—had happened by chance rather than through any plan. Performance was inconsistent, and falls were associated with patient injuries. The existing fall team was reorganized and charged with improving performance to achieve the NDNQI database best quartile performance. The FOCUS-PDSA process (Find, Organize, Clarify, Understand, Select; Plan, Do, Study, Act) and rapid cycle approach guided the work as the team reviewed the circumstances around each fall, recommended process and practice changes, and evaluated the effectiveness of those changes. (See Figure 1.)

FIGURE 1.
PDSA Model for Performance Improvement

Model for Improvement
What are we trying to accomplish?
How will we know that a change is an improvement?
What change can we make that will result in improvement?
Act
Plan
Study
Do

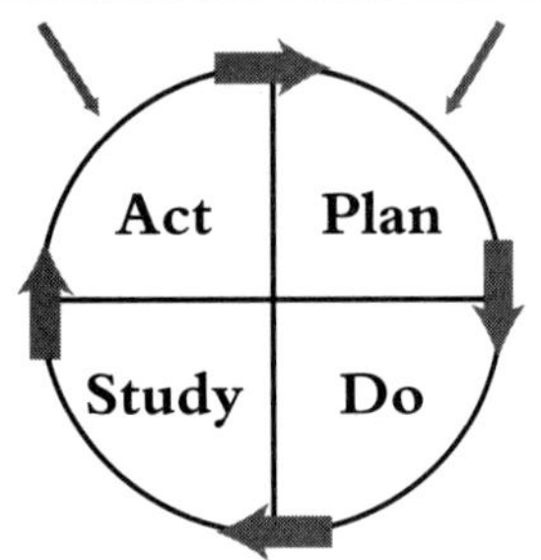

As reflected in Figure 2, process and practice changes recommended by the team resulted in an immediate decline in fall rates in the target units of CCC and MSP from Q1-06 through Q4-07. The mean fall rate of 1.25 falls per 1,000 patient days for the adult med/surg units was well below the national mean of 3.74. Performance at or near the best quartile was maintained through 2007. During the same period, falls were reduced in the inpatient rehab unit, with a December mean of 3.11 compared with the national mean of 7.24 (see Figure 3).

These results were achieved by reducing variability in patient assessment and fall prevention interventions, increasing "mindfulness" (explicit awareness), moving accountability from the hospitalwide team to the unit and from the manager to the entire staff, improving the use of technology, and identifying and resolving environmental issues. The following are considered to be the most important process and practice changes:

- Applying the rapid cycle FOCUS-PDSA process to evaluate current practice, identify evidence-based practices in fall prevention, and establish objective goals (initiated Q3-06)
- Mandating that all patients at risk of falling be attended in the bathroom (initiated Q3-06)
- Increasing staff, patient, and family mindfulness about, and accountability for, fall prevention (initiated Q3-06)
- Supervising new admissions and transfers closely the first 2 hours on the unit (initiated Q4-07)
- Changing attitudes from one of "falls happen" to "no falls will happen" (initiated Q4-07)

FIGURE 2.
Sustained Improvement in Fall Rates on Adult Med/Surg Units

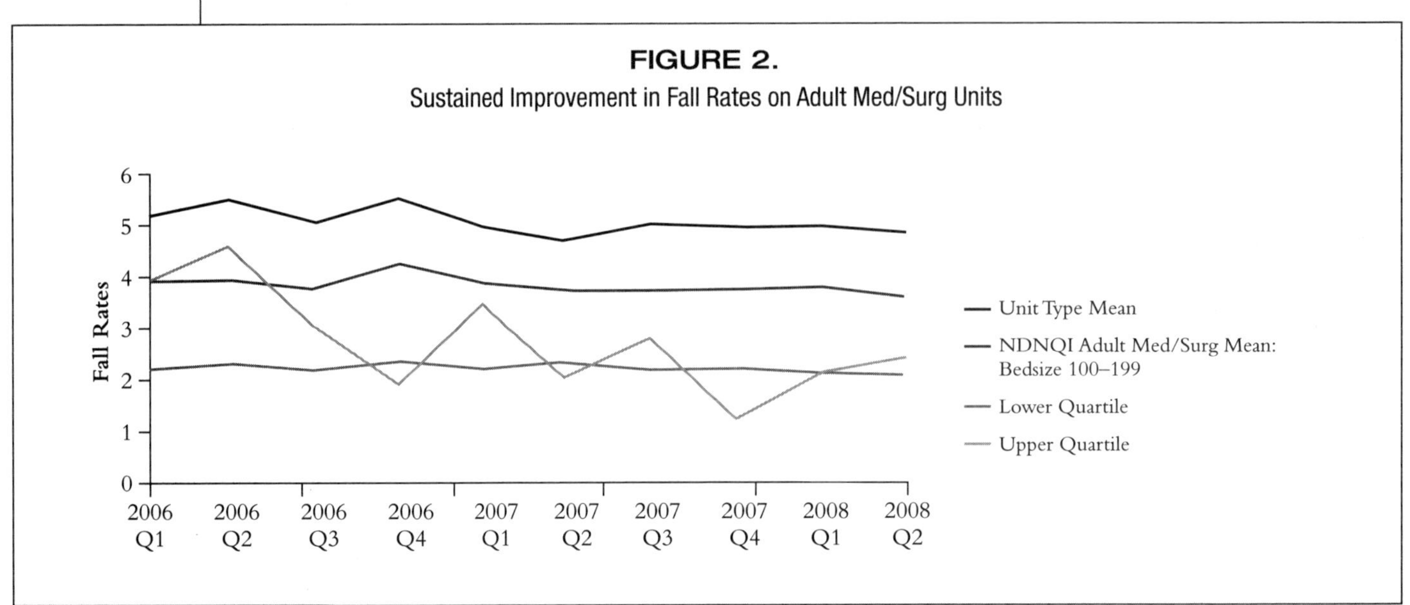

FIGURE 3.
Sustained Improvement in Fall Rates on Inpatient Rehabilitation (IPR) Unit

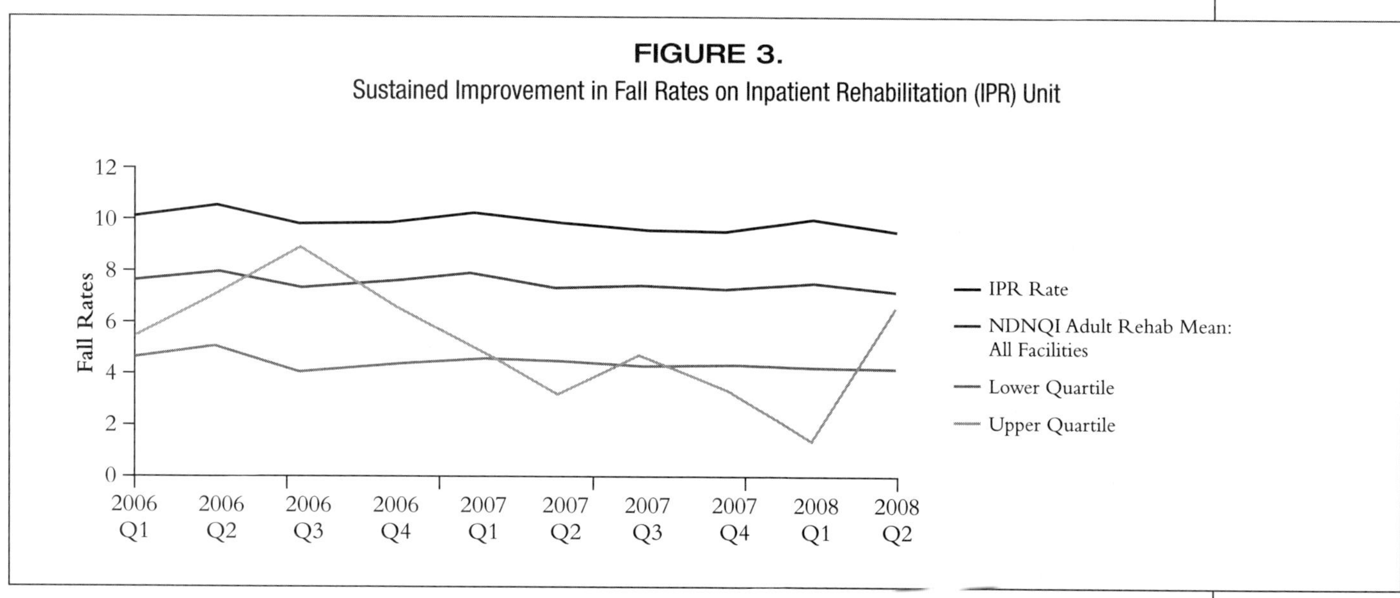

The units involved in the rapid cycle process have maintained their performance. Figure 2 reflects sustained performance on the adult medical/surgical units through Q2–08; Figure 3 reflects performance for the same period in the inpatient rehabilitation unit. RCMC has gone 616 days without a fall with a major injury. The structure and process changes that resulted in these improvements were numerous.

The RCMC Approach to Fall Prevention

Even though the fall prevention program had been a part of the RCMC nursing and patient care community since 2004, staff and leadership had developed a false sense of security with fall rates, assuming that some falls were unavoidable. The goal was to have no injury associated with a fall. Under the leadership of the director of inpatient nursing services and the manager of Inpatient Rehabilitation, the staff and leadership were challenged to look at their performance as they compared their units with other organizations in the NDNQI database. With the increase in falls and patient injury experienced by CCC, MSP, and Inpatient Rehab, staff took ownership of the opportunity to improve patient care and clinical practice. The fall team membership—a multidisciplinary group including inpatient and outpatient clinical staff and environmental services staff—was expanded to include physical therapy staff, the risk manager, and licensed and unlicensed assistive personnel from every clinical department in the hospital.

Effective September 2006, the rapid cycle FOCUS-PDSA process guided the work of the team. Rapid cycle means applying the FOCUS-PDSA process in a compressed time frame, meeting weekly to every other week, to identify, implement, and evaluate probable solutions to structure and process issues. Successful interventions were retained, while other interventions were discarded and replaced with new strategies. Immediate goals were evaluated over a 1- to 3-month period with intermediate and long-term goals providing the longer work plan extending to 18 months or longer as appropriate.

The FOCUS part of this process:

F—Find process to improve
O—Organize the team
C—Clarify the process
U—Understand indicators, root causes
S—Select and improvement

The PDSA part (see Figure 1):

P—Plan how to implement
D—Do it
S—Study the effects
A—Act on the learning and monitor gains

A literature review was conducted to identify best practices in fall risk assessment and prevention (Hendrich, 2007; Hitcho et al., 2004; Spetz, Jacobs, & Hatler, 2007; Wilson, 1998). Contacts were made with high-performing hospitals. Attention was placed on mindfulness (explicit awareness) of staff and family/patient to prevent falls, use of technology as a support, reduction of environmental causes, and staff education about fall assessment and prevention.

Staff members, serving as fall representatives for their units, conducted detailed reviews of each fall. Reviews were conducted using all assessment components in the NDNQI data reporting tool; "medication use"; cognitive and physiological patient factors; environmental factors, including use of bed exit alarms and lighting; staff knowledge about assessment and prevention; and patient knowledge of what measures to take to avoid a fall (call for assistance). The PDSA process was repeated after each measurement cycle to build on success and sustain practice changes. Appendix 1 (pp. 174–175) summarizes the FOCUS-PDSA process applied during this initiative. Additional activities included the following:

- Actions/interventions and education were provided at unit/department practice councils and monthly meetings.
- Regular reporting of opportunities and outcomes to the chief nursing officer. Individual performance issues were addressed through coaching and counseling processes and referred to the Nursing Peer Review Committee, as appropriate.
- The fall prevention plan was realigned with Joint Commission standards.
- The entire organization endorsed training and utilization of a "Just Culture" approach to addressing errors.
- All high-risk fall patients were attended at all times while in the bathroom.
- Hourly rounds were implemented, conducted by RN and unlicensed assistive personnel (UAP), to address any needs.
- Comprehensive evaluation of bed exit alarm systems was carried out, resulting in implementation of enhanced, preventive maintenance measures, staff education, and monitoring.
- Focus on falls was elevated during first 2 hours of admission or transfer.
- Staff received intense staff education on fall assessment and prevention.
- Patient safety white boards were used in staff break rooms and bathrooms stating unit-specific days since a patient fall.
- Increased engagement of patients and families was accomplished through handouts addressing their role in fall prevention and through ongoing conversation (Appendix 2, p. 175).
- Special signage was used in patient rooms identifying patients as fall risk 1, 2, or 3.
- Electronic medical record documentation was revised to facilitate assessment, risk identification, and interventions and to improve communication between caregivers.

Celebrations were conducted at the unit level with posting of "days since last fall" and verbal recognition of staff involved in fall prevention activities, and individual unit celebrations were held at unit meetings to recognize success. Outcomes were communicated to all staff via the Nursing Newsletter and at the housewide Patient Safety Committee meetings, and annually at the Quality and Safety Committee meeting of the board of directors.

How NDNQI Data Were Used in the Improvement Plan

NDNQI data provided comparison data, which were used to develop RCMC goals and assessment criteria. Each aspect of the assessment information required for NDNQI reporting was included in the assessment of causative factors. The outcomes of the hospitals performing at the best quartile in the database provided motivation to excel and validated the short-term goal of achieving performance in the top quartile and the long-term goal of achieving zero falls. The units selected were easily benchmarked using NDNQI information.

Unit Overviews

Cancer Care Center (CCC)

The Cancer Care Center provides care to inpatient geriatric patients, adults, and young adults. The major patient populations are those with medical and surgical oncology diagnoses or hematologic disorders; patients receiving chemotherapy or radiation therapy, brachytherapy, or radioactive pharmaceuticals; and stem cell transplant patients. Overflow medical and surgical patients are also part of the patient population. The staff are involved in housewide practice councils such as the Nursing Peer Review Committee, as well as unit-specific teams to address pain, falls, and transfers to a higher level of care.

Medical/Surgical Pediatrics (MSP)

MSP is a 36-bed medical, surgical, and pediatric unit with 30 medical beds and 6 pediatric beds. The unit is also telemetry capable. The unit was renamed Ortho/Neuro Peds in January 2008 when the hospital opened a new medical/surgical unit. Patient ages range from 3 days to the end of life. The goal of MSP is to provide comprehensive and evidence-based nursing care to medical, surgical, or pediatric patients. Patient types include the following:

- Pediatric patients that are newly diagnosed with type 1 diabetes, sepsis, or reactive airway disease, or infants with hyperbilirubinemia
- General medical patients with renal disease, urinary sepsis, endocrine abnormalities, abdominal symptoms
- Total joint replacement patients or patients with fractures
- All non–critical-care surgical patients, including orthopedic surgical patients
- Stable medical cardiac patients requiring telemetry assessment

Physical Rehabilitation Center (PHC)

The Physical Rehabilitation Center (PHC) at Rush-Copley Medical Center contains an 18-bed inpatient unit. Patient ages range from 18 years to end of life. The Commission for Accreditation of Rehabilitative Facilities (CARF) reviews and provides 3-year accreditation for the RCMC Physical Rehabilitation Center, which is a mark of excellence in medical rehabilitation. The physical rehabilitation department provides a full range of services, including comprehensive inpatient rehabilitation, acute hospital, and outpatient rehabilitation services. The PHC includes 24-hour nursing care, physical therapy, occupational therapy, speech therapy, recreational therapy, social services, nutritional services, spiritual services, and neuropsychological services. When possible and appropriate, outdoor community activities and outings are included to encourage patients to resume activities in the community. A board-certified physiatrist who provides overall direction of the patient's treatment plan oversees all services.

Patients may include stroke, brain injury, spinal cord injury, fractures and joint replacements, polyarthritis, amputation, Guillain-Barré, multiple sclerosis, and Parkinson's disease. Inpatient admission criteria include physical impairments that limit functional activity and potential to benefit from individualized and interdisciplinary rehabilitative services. All patients must be neurologically and medically stable, alert, and able to tolerate 3 hours of combined therapies 6 days a week.

The Consequences of Improvement

Applying the rapid cycle FOCUS-PDSA process allowed the fall team members to quickly identify the most significant process variations (causative factors) affecting patient safety related to falls. Engaging the frontline staff, consistent with the shared governance model, resulted in a commitment to quickly implement proposed solutions and evaluate their impact. The accountability to stay with patients while in the bathroom and increased awareness of risk associated with new admissions and transfers required ownership on the part of every staff person who came in contact with patients. Enculturation of that attitude and commitment is evidenced by the sustained performance and measureable outcome of *no falls with a major injury* for 616 days. The following in-house shorthand success formula captures the RCMC programmatic perspective on its fall prevention program: "Engaged staff + Leadership + Evidence-based practice + National benchmarks = SUCCESS."

Significant cost reductions occurred related to patient falls and follow-up evaluation or treatment (see Table 1). Assessment costs reflected radiology and imaging procedures conducted to determine the presence or significance of injuries with every fall that occurred. Costs decreased dramatically related to both assessment and treatment after the program was revised. Expenses for 2007 reflect costs associated with treatment related to falls with injury that occurred in 2006, *before* the fall prevention program was revised.

RCMC has achieved statewide recognition for fall reduction activities through the Illinois Hospital Association (IHA) patient safety collaborative because of the number of days without a fall with a major injury and because of the overall decrease in falls across the organization. RCMC's goal is to achieve and sustain performance at the top decile for total falls. Sustained scores on the annual RCMC employee engagement survey regarding the organizational commitment to safety ("Our environment encourages reporting medical errors and patient safety issues") also improved because of this concentration on fall safety (see Figure 4).

In 2008, the fall team was integrated into the Practice Congress for greater hospital system exposure and an ongoing commitment to frontline staff accountability for patient safety. Team members remain responsible for two-way communication with their respective units. All non-nursing areas participate on an ad hoc basis and often through task force work. Facilitation of the fall prevention conversations includes the directors for risk management and physical medicine and rehabilitation. Agendas are prepared and distributed at each meeting from work assignments made the prior month. All members have a responsibility to report at their respective unit practice congresses. The FOCUS-PDSA model continues to be used and teams are multidisciplinary.

TABLE 1.
Impact of RCMC Fall Prevention Program on Costs

FY	Cost Savings ($)	Key Driver
2006	40,000	Assessment and treatment postfall associated with minor and moderate injuries
2007	800,000	Assessment and treatment postfall associated with major and minor injuries
2008	7,000	Assessment post-fall, no injury noted

Source: Messer-Rehak, 2008.

The Illinois Hospital Association Patient Safety Collaborative has adopted RCMC's processes as best practices. Outcomes and activities since 2007 include the following:

- Continued endorsement of the fall assessment tool embedded within the current e-documentation.
- Immediate fall investigation by the director of risk management and the unit-based teams when a fall occurs, including the following: (1) the risk management director is paged or called any time, any day that a fall has occurred; (2) the staff complete their report following care to the patient; and (3) the staff notify the unit manager with follow-up documentation by the risk management director.
- A drill-down investigation, with reporting at the unit level, to the Nursing Practice Council, and to the Quality and Safety Committee of the board of directors.
- Assessment of 15-year-old medical/surgical beds for safety, including the following: (1) mattresses replaced; (2) all safety sensor strips in the beds replaced in 45 days, and annual plan developed; (3) blitz staff education undertaken for zeroing beds and activating the bed alarms, and for troubleshooting bed problems; and (4) recommendation made to the administrative team to expedite bed replacement through the capital program, with 45 beds replaced in calendar year 2008.
- Organizational philosophical shift to "There will be zero falls at our facility."
- Patients at highest fall level (level 3) to use bedside commode during night shift for toileting.
- Staff scripting to encourage patient and families to call for assistance in the room or bathroom.
- Coaching to staff about balancing patient satisfaction with keeping the patients safe.
- Ongoing assessment of the fall prevention plan against best practice standards such as the Agency for Healthcare Research and Quality and the Illinois Hospital Association's Patient Safety Collaborative.

FIGURE 4.
Employee Engagement Survey Reflecting Organizational Commitment to Safety

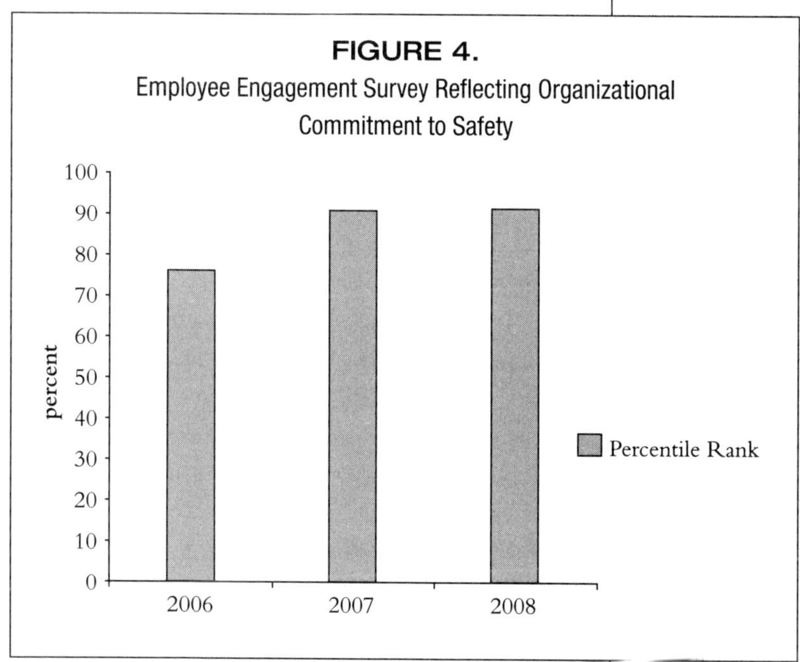

- Hospitalwide implementation of patient safety ambassadors for each nursing area: (1) to monitor and assess safety in their respective areas, (2) to facilitate conversations to enhance the patient environment with other departments, and (3) to facilitate safety conversations during their unit-based practice meetings.
- Implementation of safety white boards in nursing unit staff areas that document "the number of days since a patient with a [fall, unit acquired pressure ulcer, or employee lift] injury." These boards are maintained daily by the unit patient safety ambassador or the designee and are to be reviewed during staffing huddles, information hand-off, and unit-based meetings.

The RCMC Approach to Fall Prevention: Conclusion and Implications

Engaging staff and leadership was the first step in creating the synergy needed to improve performance. A key to that engagement was objectively identifying the opportunity for improvement by evaluating the impact of RCMC's performance on patients and con-

TABLE 2.
Fall Safety-Related Expenditures

Item	Cost
Replacement of safety sensor strips, 2/bed, for 138 beds	$100,000
Stocking with additional replacement strips for 3 years	$98,000
Staff education completed by managers and nurse educators	$3,000
3-year bed replacement plan without leases	$2,400,000

firming that the center could do better, as evidenced by other successful organizations. The NDNQI database provided the performance measures that RCMC strove to achieve, as well as a starting point for the issues to review as contributing factors.

Having administrative support reinforced the importance of fall prevention. The chief nursing officer and the directors and managers of these units supported staff by assuming the role of fall prevention advocates and by providing time to conduct evaluations and staff education. Additional administrative support included funds to replace or repair bed exit alarms, educate staff, and support an accelerated plan for replacement of med/surg beds over 3 years (Table 2). The original bed replacement plan was reduced from a 5-year plan to a 3-year plan because of the perceived impact on patient safety (Hitcho et al., 2004: Spetz et al., 2007).

Staff actively collaborated with the risk manager to conduct a focused review of each fall to identify trends in contributing factors and to develop a corrective action plan using a rapid cycle FOCUS-PDSA approach. The nurses at the bedside were the ones reinforcing all the practice changes and celebrating successes with their colleagues. They used evidence-based practice changes identified through literature searches and contact with best-performing organizations. Staff engaged non-nursing staff, unlicensed assistive personnel, and other clinicians and nonclinical support staff to assist in fall assessment and prevention and to respond to bed exit alarms, ensuring a quick response time to prevent falls. They established the expectation and monitored compliance with attending at-risk patients in the bathroom, the focus on new admissions and transfers, and the attitudinal change that all falls are preventable.

Staff also recommended using the formal structure of the Nursing Peer Review Committee to reinforce professional accountability and autonomy in a non-punitive manner by using a panel of peer experts to critique and guide practice. The literature reviewed by the fall team did not identify accessing the formal nursing peer review structure as a strategy to increase individual accountability and frontline staff involvement in problem identification. The process of referring individual cases for review to a panel of peers (nursing peer review) is believed to foster individual accountability and professional practice in a less punitive approach. It accomplishes this by having peers first review the circumstances around an occurrence and then communicate directly with the staff involved in the case to problem solve and educate.

The role of shared governance in sustaining RCMC's outcomes was crucial. The Practice Congress, composed of staff nurses from all departments, reinforced the cultural change to maintain individual accountability. The congress also implemented the accountability model that ensured that the recommendations from the fall team would be implemented to demonstrate the individual professional accountability for performance and the commitment to patient safety that was sought from employees. Additional lessons learned are described in Table 3.

The impact on patient care is clearly demonstrated by the fact that RCMC has achieved 616 days without a fall with a major injury. RCMC staff members are more confident about organizational commitment to patient safety and have significantly reduced costs associated with patient assessment and treatment following a fall. By applying this formula for success, the RCMC fall team has maintained all of the activities that have been identified as key to preventing falls:

- Attendance for all high-risk patients while in the bathrooms, to reduce the risk of falls.
- Addition of chair-check alarms to notify staff of patient position changes.
- Patient and family education related to fall safety, upon admission, and notification of staff for needed assistance (see Appendix 2, p. 175).
- Policy and procedure development related to fall reduction and documentation.
- Patient assessment using an electronic fall assessment tool that included scoring and recommendations for staff interventions to reduce fall risk.
- Use of door signage and colored armbands to identify patients at risk of falling.
- Development of transport passes to provide timely information between units and areas in the hospital.
- Hourly patient rounding by nursing and clinical aid staff for safety, toileting, pain management, and connection with the patient and family.

Over the next 24 months, the team will plan and implement a research study incorporating the NDNQI assessment information, the RCMC fall assessment tool, and the risk factors on admission, and any time a fall occurs will determine what key predictors can be identified specific to the RCMC patient population. The team will then explore what interventions may have made a difference based on the key predictors and will use that to guide RCMC's fall prevention program.

TABLE 3.
RCMC Lessons Learned in Fall Prevention

- It is challenging to keep momentum and focus on fall prevention.
- It is extremely challenging to achieve "mindfulness" or ongoing staff awareness related to safety for novice RNs or support staff, along with their other responsibilities.
- Bed exit alarms do not prevent falls; they only notify staff if a patient changes positions.
- Celebration provides energy for future successes.
- Flexibility is needed with modes of staff education to enhance the learning process, including:
  - Classroom—Orientation
  - Electronic—Orientation, didactic, relearning
  - Unit-based—One-on-one or small group, competency, or process change
  - Just-in-time—By topic experts, unit educators, or competencied staff
- E-mail—Reminders, follow through with activities or time-sensitive learnings.
- If trends cannot be found, then keep digging!

References

Hendrich, A. (2007). Predicting patient falls. *American Journal of Nursing, 107*(11), 50–58.

Hitcho, E. B., Krauss, M. J., Birge, S., Dunagan, W. C., Fischer, I., Johnson, S., et al. (2004). Characteristics and circumstances of falls in a hospital setting. *Journal of General Internal Medicine, 19,* 732–739.

Messer-Rehak, D. (2008). *Internal cost comparative analysis related to costs associated with falls.* Aurora, IL.

Spetz, J., Jacobs, J., & Hatler, C. (2007). Cost effectiveness of a medical vigilance system to reduce patient falls. *Nursing Economics, 25*(6), 333–338.

Wilson, E. B. (1998). Preventing patient falls. *AACN Clinical Issues, 9*(1): 100–108.

Background Resources

Boat, T. F., Chao, S. M., & O'Neill, P. H. (2008). From waste to value in healthcare. *Journal of the American Medical Association, 299*(5), 568–570.

Centers for Disease Control and Prevention. (2008). Self-reported falls and fall-related injuries among persons aged >65 years. *United States, Morbidity and Mortality Weekly Report, 57*(9), 225–229.

Illinois Hospital Association. (2008). *Comparison data from hospitals participating in the Patient Safety Collaborative.* Naperville, IL: Author.

The Joint Commission. (2006, 2007, 2008). *National patient safety goals.* Retrieved January 9, 2009, from http://www.jointcommission.org.

Appendix 1. RCMC Fall Reduction Strategy—Initial FOCUS-PDSA, conducted September 2006

Find: Opportunity/need to reduce the number of preventable patient falls with/without injury to better than the national benchmark of the NDQI database in CCC, MSP (renamed Ortho/Neuro Peds in Jan. 2008, or ONP), and PHC units.

Organize: Work team composed of inpatient nursing staff, the director of the inpatient units, the manager of the Physical Rehabilitation Center, a nursing clinical analyst, facilities management, and the hospital risk manager reporting to the nursing Practice Congress and Performance Improvement Council.

Clarify: Current knowledge of the process and make immediate improvements. Prepare a flow chart of the current process and identify immediate opportunities for improvement.

Understand: *Sources of process variation are the primary causative factors associated with falls:*

Current fall assessment and fall prevention strategies vary from unit to unit and shift to shift:

- Applying fall risk definitions and rates vary.
- Documentation and communication of fall risk status are inconsistent or absent.
- Use of bed alarm equipment varies and functionality is not assessed or maintained consistently.
- Hands-off communication does not consistently address risk level or preventive measures that are in place.
- Accountability is placed on the housewide committee or the manager rather than the individual practitioner.
- Staff attitude is one of accepting that falls will happen rather than one of believing that all falls can be prevented and should not happen to hospitalized patients.

Measures that reflect improvement in process variation include: *Number of falls per unit.*

Patient identification band and signage on the door indicate fall risk score for the patient.

Select: Communication of process changes.

Identify: Time frames for completing fall risk assessment and documentation.

- Monthly audits of patients at risk for fall as determined by the fall assessments.
- Mandatory education.
- Unit projects to evaluate products and procedures.
- Mandatory attendance during toileting to reduce preventable bathroom falls by 50% in 3 months.

Provide: Monthly feedback to units on number of falls and findings of peer review.

Plan: Under fall team leadership, evaluate each fall that occurs on the three target units (CCC, MSP/ONP, and Inpatient Rehab) within 1 business day using NDNQI process questions supplemented with specific concerns identified by RCMC team. Staff seeking career ladder advancement and unit-based nurses who are members of the Nursing Peer Review Committee will be involved in the evaluations.

- Fall team members present initial unit-specific findings of audits and review of past 2 months of falls.
- Instruct all staff on rounding and attending patients in bathroom.

Do: Implement on three inpatient units; complete focused fall assessments; propose, implement, and evaluate solutions; revise based on outcomes; educate via online computer-based learning modules (PowerPoint and educational videos with test questions) and learning modules posters, presentations at unit meetings, and posters on each unit identifying "days without falls."

Study: Outcomes reported monthly to fall team and Practice Congress, quarterly to Patient Safety Committee, annually to Board.

Act: Reinforce all measures that reduce falls; develop additional interventions based on contributing factors identified with focused review.

Repeat PDSA cycle monthly until target is achieved.

Appendix 2. Patient and Family Education Material

A Note About Patient Safety and Fall Prevention

A fall is defined as "any unplanned or uncontrolled descent to the floor, with or without injury incurred."

At Rush-Copley Medical Center we believe all patients have the right to be cared for in a safe environment. Our goal is to accomplish this without the risk of falls.

The registered nurse (RN) will screen and monitor all patients upon admission to the medical center, and every 8 hours throughout their stay to determine their risk for falls. Examples might include:

- Make sure the call light is within reach and encourage the patient to call.
- Apply fall prevention orange wristband and explain patient is at risk to fall.
- Use bed and chair monitor alarms to alert staff.
- Do frequent staff rounding to check patient and offer toileting.
- Give patient nonskid footwear.
- Use side rails.
- Never leave high-risk patient unattended while up to bathroom or ambulating.

Instructions to the Family

- Advise the nurse of any condition patient has that may affect balance or ability to ambulate independently.
- Never turn off the bed or chair alarm, or lower the side rails without nursing staff present to assist patient.
- Know how to use the call light.

Afterword: The Importance of Comparing the Costs and Effects of Quality Improvement

Kevin D. Frick, PhD
Johns Hopkins Bloomberg School of Public Health

The chapters in this monograph focus on nurse satisfaction, nurse certification and education, pressure ulcer prevention, and falls prevention. Most of the chapters describe interventions with a focus on organizational readiness for change. The chapters describe the challenges and successes that different hospitals experienced.

Few chapters have included information on costs. The chapter describing the education initiative at the Shea Campus of Scottsdale Healthcare had a clear focus on costs. Costs are an important part of any organizational decision to invest in quality improvement. Costs can (1) be critical for budgeting; (2) inform a cost–consequence analysis in which the costs are juxtaposed with a variety of effects of the intervention; (3) inform a comparison of the total costs and monetary benefits to facilitate an assessment of the return on investment in quality improvement; (4) inform a cost-effectiveness analysis that provides a structured method of calculating a "unit price of better health" by comparing data on the costs of an intervention with data on the primary clinical outcomes of the intervention; and (5) provide a context for considering how the intervention changes the production of care and changes the hospital's profitability as a result. Each of these will be discussed in turn, along with a commentary on the sources of cost data to facilitate each type of analysis.

Budgeting

Costs are an obvious necessity for budgeting purposes. While the need for some changes may be dictated by a need to maintain or improve quality, changes that are more elective likely will be made only if they are deemed to yield a reasonable return on investment. Even if no formal return-on-investment analysis is done, decision-makers (including nurse managers and administrators at all levels) will need to know how much the intervention will cost to be able to budget for intervention activities.

Concepts

When considering the resources necessary and the costs that will be calculated, we can divide them into three sections. First, the intervention may have start-up costs that will be the same regardless of how long the intervention goes on and how large the intervention may eventually become. Since the resources cannot be changed once the intervention has begun, they can also be referred to as *sunk costs*. Since these costs do not vary with the eventual size of the program, they can be referred to as *fixed costs*. The term fixed costs can also be used to describe costs that are recurring (rather than only experienced at start-up) but that are the same regardless of the program's size.

An example of start-up costs will help to clarify the terminology. Consider a novel nurse orientation program that is designed to improve nurse job satisfaction, and that will begin in a single unit and then expand if the single unit intervention is successful. Sunk costs will be those associated with the orientation of the first cohort of nurses who receive the orientation in the unit initiating the program. The costs that are specific to the first unit include curriculum development, associated materials, and the development of new procedures. If the nurse manager and other administrators cannot project the sunk costs, the program will need to be initiated with very little information for budgeting; this would seem unlikely to occur. However, even when the sunk costs can be predicted, these will affect the budget only once.

The term *fixed costs* most commonly refers to costs that are fixed but recurring. These were mentioned above and contrasted with sunk costs, the fixed one-time-only costs. An example of fixed but recurring costs will help to clarify terminology. If there is an administrator who has to dedicate time to the novel orientation process regardless of how many nurses get trained each year, then the administrator's time would be an ongoing fixed cost. In contrast, while the development of materials was a sunk cost, the printing of new materials for the orientation of each new cohort of nurses in each additional unit is not sunk and is not even fixed. The additional materials for each new orientation fall into the next category discussed below.

The third category of costs, *variable costs*, includes those that depend on the size of the program. In the hypothetical nurse orientation program, the orientation costs vary with the number of nurses in the unit, that is, the number of nurses needing to receive the orientation or reorientation. The costs of expanding the program to other units also are variable from the perspective of the program initiation. Both are examples of costs that have to be budgeted each year.

Data

Having identified the different types of costs as sunk, other fixed, or variable costs, the question for any nurse manager planning to collect cost data becomes: where are the data to be found? Costs are a function of the quantities of the resources that are required and the price of each of those resources. While expenditure data may be the most easily obtained, particularly for monitoring the costs for future budgeting, the initial budgeting process requires separate figures on the quantities of resources and the associated prices. Even moving forward from the initial budgeting process—separating the calculation into quantities and prices rather than simply using expenditures—can be useful for a variety of reasons. Most important, understanding possible variation in the costs is aided most by understanding the quantities and prices separately. When there are separate data on quantities and prices, it is easier to examine the potential effects of hiring more nurses, as distinguished from the effects of paying nurses higher wages.

Expenditure data would likely come from reports that a nurse manager or other administrator is required to submit or from cost accounting reports that are developed from a hospital's or health system's finance department. Obtaining expenditure data may be easier than obtaining data on specific quantities of resources being used. The finance department will necessarily have data on prices. The quantities may be difficult to assess because a hospital or other work environment often knows the total that was paid to a nurse but does not track specifically every moment that the nurse spends performing different tasks. For the hypothetical orientation program, a deliberate decision would be required to collect data on attendance at the orientation meetings and the time spent at orientation meetings. An additional deliberate decision would need to be made to collect data on all copies of materials, all binders, and all food service. The same would be true for any other program or intervention. The key is that tracking resources used at the detailed level of the specific intervention or program is not necessarily a standard function of the nurse manager's job. Making a deliberate decision to collect these data is required to understand the separate implications of price changes and program size changes or of price changes for different resources that are required.

Using the Cost Data to Make Comparisons: Cost–Consequence Analysis

Nurse managers and other administrators faced with decisions about whether to implement specific quality improvement interventions or programs may want to know more than simply the cost of the intervention. The earlier chapters in this monograph have reported on the successes and challenges of different quality improvement initiatives. Analyzing the changes brought about by the initiatives and the cost of the initiatives is referred to as a cost–consequence analysis. This is rather straightforward as it simply involves describing the costs attributable to the initiative and all consequences of the initiative. The consequences can be either positive (cost savings or improved nurse satisfaction) or negative (additional costs or nurses feeling like one more orientation program is a waste of time). The consequences can be immediate or traced to their long-run implications. The consequences of multiple initiatives could be compared and contrasted with the costs of the different initiatives. In other words, if a nurse manager is considering multiple ways by which the job satisfaction of the nursing staff can be improved, the different costs and consequences can be compared. This essentially is making a list of the pros and cons of different initiatives for further consideration in the decision-making process, including the cost data.

The ease of a cost–consequence analysis is that the consequences can be described simply as they occur. The difficulty with this type of analysis is that it is not obvious how much it should cost to improve by 10 percentage points, for example, the proportion of nurses who describe the day as a good one and the proportion of physicians who are more satisfied with their working relationships with the nurses. The same can be true of other measures of nurse satisfaction and measures of personnel interaction. Without having a clear idea of what it should cost to achieve multiple positive outcomes (or having a mixture of positive and negative outcomes), a nurse manager will simply need to justify to herself or himself and to the other administrators that the expenditures can be considered worthwhile.

Budget Impact Analysis

While a reading of the cost-related literature reveals that different analysts take different perspectives (that is, taking the point of view of different stakeholders) in conducting their analyses, most nurse managers work within a healthcare system or for a hospital for which the primary concern is its own bottom line. In this case, the next step following an assessment of the costs of a quality improvement initiative would be the measurement of and the application of a monetary value to the effects or benefits of the initiative. The chapters discussing the efforts to reduce pressure ulcers or falls provide good examples of the need for and usefulness of budget impact analyses.

These analyses require that the manager understand the effects of the intervention in terms of the reduced number of falls or the reduced rate of hospital acquired pressure ulcers and understand the financial impact of each fall or pressure ulcer for the hospital. The changes that occur in the clinical outcome must be monitored carefully and measured in ways that clearly demonstrate that the changes are a result of the quality improvement initiative. This, of course, is already the focus of the chapters of this monograph. The key is that the financial implications of each change must also be understood.

Whether the nurse manager is looking at only the costs for the hospital or health system or is considering broader cost implications (for example, the patient and family costs associated with a fall) of the clinical changes, this type of analysis can be referred to as a cost–benefit analysis, in addition to being referred to as a budget impact analysis. The notion here is that a direct comparison can be made between the monetary costs and benefits of a program. Budget impact analysis is useful because it provides a direct way of comparing the magnitudes. This type of analysis can be challenging because understanding even the average financial implications of a fall or pressure ulcer is not trivial.

Cost-Effectiveness

In some cases obtaining the data on the changes in outcomes is straightforward, but it is not as simple to obtain data on the monetary value associated with those outcomes. In this case, rather than summarizing the results of the quality improvement initiative in a budget impact or cost–benefit analysis, the nurse manager and other administrators can consider the results as summarized in a cost-effectiveness analysis. Such an analysis compares the changes in cost associated with a new quality improvement initiative or the difference in costs between quality improvement initiatives with the changes in a single outcome. The key is that there is a single outcome or some way of summarizing all outcomes in a single measure. This gives us the opportunity to discuss the unit cost of improvements, and this works only when there is a summary outcome. For nurse satisfaction it could be a comparison of costs with the percentage of nurses responding that the day was good overall. While this is generally a useful summary measure, it may also be the case that because nurse satisfaction has the potential to be a highly multidimensional measure, a manager may want to maintain the cost–consequence analysis approach in this case to capture those different dimensions.

For the quality improvement initiatives aimed at reducing hospital acquired pressure ulcers or falls, the obvious summary outcome is the incidence of pressure ulcers or falls. The key here is that everyone can agree that it is useful to ask how much extra it might cost to provide care while avoiding a pressure ulcer or a fall. The difficulty is that not everyone will necessarily agree on how much the hospital or health system should be willing to spend to avoid such outcomes. Similar to the situation of cost–consequence analysis, in this case the nurse manager will have to justify that the spending is worthwhile. However, this process is simpler than cost–consequence analysis because there is a single clearly defined and agreed-upon outcome metric.

Economics and Costs

Most hospitals have an incentive for providing care of a given quality at the minimum cost of production. To the degree that the hospital can set its own prices, those prices will be related to the cost of production. Having an understanding of the costs of a particular quality improvement will allow the nurse manager and other administrators to make decisions that minimize costs. A hospital's financial survival is not guaranteed by cost-minimizing behavior, and some hospitals may have objectives that extend beyond cost minimization. However, a hospital's financial survival can be seriously hampered when thought is not given to maintaining and improving efficiency of operations. For not-for-profit teaching hospitals, in particular, there may be many other goals that must be considered. The key is to understand the place of efficiency and the way in which data on costs can help to improve efficiency.

Summary

Nurse managers considering a variety of possible quality improvement initiatives will need to prioritize taking the steps involved in each initiative, over not doing so, and likely will need to prioritize among the initiatives at some point. Knowing the positive impacts and challenges of each initiative is a critical step in the prioritization process. However, without a clear sense of the costs of the programs, the prioritization process will be incomplete.

One of the chapters in the monograph has already described the costs of the quality improvement initiative. Tracking costs of tuition and other educational assistance is fairly straightforward because the allocation is likely to occur on a case-by-case basis for which a decision on each nurse's interest in educational training is recorded. Tracking costs for other programs may be more complex.

Nurse managers who understand the concepts of sunk, fixed, and variable cost; how the data to calculate such costs can be collected; and the juxtaposition of costs and effects in the prioritization process will be better able to contribute to organizational decisions to enhance quality as efficiently as possible. This brief discussion illuminates those points. However, this is only the start of a process to understand and be able to use the tools that have been described. There are entire lectures or courses in schools of nursing, in related programs in schools of public health or business schools, and at professional conferences that can expand a manager's knowledge about the tools and the methods necessary to implement them. In a time of increasingly scarce resources, nurse managers are likely to find it increasingly useful and perhaps even necessary to avail themselves of opportunities to learn more about these tools so that they can become part of the toolkit that is available for making decisions and persuading others of the logic behind such decisions.

Appendix A. National Database of Nursing Quality Indicators[1]

Quarterly Nursing-Sensitive Indicators[2, 3]

- Catheter-Associated Urinary Tract Infections* (CAUTI)
- Central Line-Associated Blood Stream Infections* (CLABSI)
- Nursing Hours per Patient Day*
  - Registered Nurses (RN)
  - Licensed Practical/Vocational Nurses (LPN/LVN)
  - Unlicensed Assistive Personnel (UAP)
- Patient Falls*
- Patient Falls with Injury*
  - Injury Level
- Pediatric Pain Assessment, Intervention, Reassessment (AIR) Cycle
- Pediatric Peripheral IV Infiltration (PIV)
- Percent of Total Nursing Hours Supplied by Agency Staff*
- Pressure Ulcers
  - Total
  - Hospital Acquired
  - Unit Acquired
- Psychiatric Physical/Sexual Assault Rate
- Restraint Prevalence*
- RN Education & Certification
- Turnover
  - Voluntary Turnover* (adapted from NQF for the unit level)
  - Magnet™ Controllable Turnover
  - Total Turnover
- Skill Mix*—Percent of Total Nursing Hours Supplied by:
  - RNs
  - LPN/LVNs
  - UAPs
- Ventilator-Acquired Pneumonia* (VAP)

RN Survey Measures[3,4]

There are two primary versions of the survey. The first contains Job Satisfaction Scales (A) while the second contains the Practice Environment Scales (B). Both versions contain all of the items (C through E).

A. Job Satisfaction Scales

- NDNQI-Adapted Index of Work Satisfaction
  - Task
  - Nurse–Nurse Interactions
  - Nurse–Physician Interactions
  - Decision-Making
  - Autonomy
  - Professional Status
  - Pay
- NDNQI Adapted Nursing Work Index
  - Nurse Management
  - Nursing Administration
  - Professional Development
- Selected Individual-level Job Satisfaction Items

B. Practice Environment Scale of the Nursing Work Index

- Nurse Participation in Hospital Affairs
- Nursing Foundations for Quality of care
- Nurse Manager Ability
- Leadership and Support of Nurses
- Staffing and Resource Adequacy
- Collegial Nurse–Physician relations

C. Job Enjoyment Scale

D. Work Contextual Items

- RN Job Plans for Next Year
- Unit Quality of Care
- Unit Orientation
- Hospital Recommendation
- Description of Unit Last Shift
- Situations on Unit Last Shift
- Meal Breaks on Unit Last Shift
- Non-Meal Breaks on Unit Last Shift
- Hours Worked by Units RNs Last Shift
- Usual Shift and Rotation of Unit RNs
- Floating of Unit RNs
- Unit RNs Working Extra Hours
- Unit Acuity and Staffing

E. RN Characteristics

- Average Unit RN Gender, Race, Age, Role and Job Situation
- Average Unit RN Tenure
- Average Unit RN Education
- Average Unit RN Certification

* National Quality Forum (NQF) Consensus Standard

1. Visit NDNQI's web site: www.nursingquality.org for more information. Measures are Structure, Process, and Outcomes based on Donabedian's Quality Framework.

2. All indicators are collected and reported quarterly.

3. Comparison reports with national data are provided for categories of all hospitals, bed size, teaching status, Magnet™ status, hospital type, census divisions, case mix index, metropolitan status and selected adult unit specialties. Data are reported by unit type.

4. Collected and reported annually.

Appendix B. National Quality Forum Indicators

Table 1.
National Voluntary Consensus Standards for Nursing-Sensitive Care

Framework Category	Measure	Description
Patient-centered outcome measures	1. Death among surgical inpatients with treatable serious complications (failure to rescue)	Percentage of major surgical inpatients who experience a hospital-acquired complication (i.e., sepsis, pneumonia, gastrointestinal bleeding, shock/cardiac arrest, deep vein thrombosis/pulmonary embolism) and die
	2. Pressure ulcer prevalence	Percentage of inpatients who have a hospital acquired pressure ulcer (Stage 2 or greater)
	3. Falls prevalence	Number of inpatient falls per inpatient days
	4. Falls with injury	Number of inpatient falls with injuries per inpatient days
	5. Restraint prevalence (vest and limb only)	Percentage of inpatients who have a vest or limb restraint
	6. Urinary catheter-associated urinary tract infection (UTI) for intensive care unit (ICU) patients	Rate of UTI associated with use of urinary catheters for ICU patients
	7. Central line catheter-associated blood stream infection rate for ICU and high-risk nursery (HRN) patients	Rate of blood stream infections associated with use of central line catheters for ICU and HRN patients
	8. Ventilator associated pneumonia for ICU and HRN patients	Rate of pneumonia associated with use of ventilators for ICU patients and HRN patients
Nursing-centered intervention measures	9. Smoking cessation counseling for acute myocardial infarction (AMI)	Percentage of AMI inpatients with history of smoking within the past year who received smoking cessation advice or counseling during hospitalization
	10. Smoking cessation counseling for heart failure (HF)	Percentage of HF inpatients with history of smoking within the past year who received smoking cessation advice or counseling during hospitalization
	11. Smoking cessation counseling for pneumonia	Percentage of pneumonia inpatients with history of smoking within the past year who received smoking cessation advice or counseling during hospitalization

TABLE 1.
National Voluntary Consensus Standards for Nursing-Sensitive Care, Continued

Framework Category	Measure	Description
System-centered measures	12. Skill mix (registered nurse [RN], licensed vocational/practical nurse [LVN/LPN], unlicensed assistive personnel [UAP], and contract)	• Percentage of RN care hours to total nursing care hours • Percentage of LVN/LPN care hours to total nursing care hours • Percentage of UAP care hours to total nursing care hours • Percentage of contract hours (RN, LVN/LPN, and UAP) to total nursing care hours
	13. Nursing care hours per patient day (RN, LVN/LPN, and UAP)	• Number of RN care hours per patient day • Number of nursing staff hours (RN, LVN/LPN, UAP) per patient day
	14. Practice Environment Scale—Nursing Work Index (PES-NWI) (composite and five subscales)	Composite score and mean presence scores for each of the following subscales derived from the PES-NWI: • Nurse participation in hospital affairs • Nursing foundations for quality of care • Nurse manager ability, leadership, and support of nurses • Staffing and resource adequacy • Collegial nurse–physician relations
	15. Voluntary turnover	Number of voluntary, uncontrolled separations during the month for RNs and advanced practice nurses, LVN/LPNs, and nurse assistants/aides

Source: National Quality Forum (2004). National Consensus Standards for Nursing Sensitive Care: An initial performance measure set. Washington, DC: National Quality Forum. Page 14. Reproduced with permission.

Note: Some of these indicators are being reviewed and are likely to be updated during 2009. Visit http://www.qualityforum.org/nursing/ to remain informed about the current status of these NQF indicators.